DATE DUE

DEC 1 4 2004	
JAN 1 1 2005	
JAN 22 2005	
FEB 06 2005	

DEMCO, INC. 38-2931

AUG 3 0 2004

MODERN MEDICINES

MODERN MEDICINES: The Discovery and Development of Healing Drugs

Facts On File, Inc.
132 West 31st Street
New York NY 10001

Library of Congress Cataloging-in-Publication Data
Facklam, Margery.
Modern medicines : the discovery and development of healing drugs /
Margery Facklam, Howard Facklam, and Sean M. Grady.
p. cm.—(Science and technology in focus)
Includes bibliographical references and index.
ISBN 0-8160-4706-5 (hc.)
1. Pharmacology—History. 2. Pharmacology. I. Facklam, Howard. II. Grady,
Sean M., 1965–III. Title. IV. Science & technology in focus
RM41.F33 2003
615′.1′09—dc21   2003011489

Facts On File books are available at special discounts when purchased in bulk quantities for businesses, associations, institutions, or sales promotions. Please call our Special Sales Department in New York at (212) 967-8800 or (800) 322-8755.

You can find Facts On File on the World Wide Web at http://www.factsonfile.com

Text design by Erika K. Arroyo
Cover design by Nora Wertz
Illustrations by Sholto Ainslie

Printed in the United States of America

MP Hermitage 10 9 8 7 6 5 4 3 2 1

This book is printed on acid-free paper.

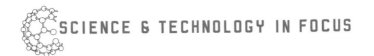

SCIENCE & TECHNOLOGY IN FOCUS

MODERN MEDICINES

The Discovery and Development
of Healing Drugs

Margery Facklam,
Howard Facklam, and
Sean M. Grady

☑®

Facts On File, Inc.

CONTENTS

ACKNOWLEDGMENTS

The authors wish to thank all those who provided information and photographs for *Modern Medicines*, the revised edition of the 1992 book *Healing Drugs: The History of Pharmacology*. In particular, they wish to thank Lisa Bayne of the Eli Lilly and Company archives; Pat Virgil and Linda Kennedy of the Buffalo & Erie County Historical Society; and John Swann of the U.S. Food and Drug Administration.

Special thanks also to Frank K. Darmstadt, Executive Editor, and Cynthia Yazbek, Associate Editor, for their forbearance with its preparation.

INTRODUCTION

Whether through great epidemics such as the Black Death that killed more than one-quarter of the population of Europe—roughly 40 million people—in the 14th century or through infections of wounds as simple as the scratch from a rosebush, disease has been a constant companion of humanity.

While all but a rare few of us are born with immune systems that adequately protect against many diseases, our immune systems often fail to withstand the assault by bacteria, viruses, molds, parasites, and other microscopic threats called pathogens that are around and within us all the time. At these times, we can turn to modern medicine: antibiotics to fight off bacteria, fungi, and even some forms of cancer; painkillers such as aspirin and ibuprofen, which also help fight fever and inflammation; antihistamines that short-circuit the symptoms of hay fever and other allergies. Using these and other healing drugs has helped many people gain the upper hand over disease and has freed them from much of the fear and helplessness they might feel when confronted with disease.

In the past, death from illness was a common part of life. Childhood was an especially dangerous time, when germs easily could overwhelm a boy's or a girl's still-developing immune system. Many children died before reaching their teen years, though adulthood did not guarantee freedom from illness. Old age was equally dangerous, leaving men and women as vulnerable to death from infections as their grandchildren.

One of the most upsetting aspects of disease was the lack of an easily identified cause. Few people knew, or even suspected, that microscopic organisms were to blame for disease until nearly the end of the 19th century. Noxious gases, imbalances in a person's body fluids, eating the wrong type of food at the wrong time of year, witchcraft—these were the explanations common folk and professional healers came up with to explain the outbreak of illness.

The remedies they relied on also varied widely—using herbs and other plants, taking part in healing rituals, wearing talismans that supposedly had the power to turn away evil spirits of disease. Some were, from a modern perspective, truly absurd. One treatment given to a European king in the Middle Ages was a concoction of crushed pearls and gemstones mixed in a goblet of wine. Drinking the mixture was supposed to infuse the patient with the "magical powers" of the gems. In truth, the only likely effect the potion had was to give the royal patient a stomachache.

Other remedies, though, turned out to have true medical benefits. Scientific examination of an ancient European remedy for headaches, tea made from the bark of a willow tree, led to the discovery of aspirin. Likewise, investigating a cure for malaria used by Indians in the mountains of Peru—the powdered bark of the cinchona tree—resulted in the discovery of quinine, an effective fever medicine as well as a reliable means of treating the disease.

Nevertheless, diseases of all sorts caused devastation around the globe until well into the 20th century. For example, a worldwide outbreak, or pandemic, of the Spanish flu in 1918 and 1919 killed so many people that their numbers are still disputed to this day. Conservative figures from the early 1920s indicated a total of 21 million deaths. More recent estimates place the toll near 40 million—four times as many deaths as had been caused during the four years of World War I, which ended shortly after the first signs of the pandemic appeared.

With the discovery that bacteria, viruses, and other pathogens caused diseases came a revolution in the way diseases were studied and treated. Events such as the Spanish flu pandemic prompted medical researchers to find new ways to attack these invisible invaders within the human body. Penicillin, tetracycline, and other antibiotics came about as the result of this research. At the same time, researchers began expanding upon the technique of vaccination, which was developed in the 18th century by an English physician as a means of combating smallpox. The widespread eradication of polio, a crippling disease that can leave its victims partially paralyzed, and the virtual elimination of smallpox from the world are just two of the technique's most astounding successes.

These and other medical developments, together with the demand for the drugs that have been created, made the medical drug industry the richest single sector of the modern global economy. More than telecommunications, computers, or even agriculture, pharmaceuticals (the collective term for medical drugs) are in such high demand that large, established firms and small start-ups alike are in constant full-throttle competition to bring new drugs to market. Many nations have developed an intricate—and, some manufacturers and physicians say, overbearing—system of regulations to qualify drugs for use and to remove drugs that turn out to cause more harm than good.

The development of modern pharmaceuticals has not been a simple matter, though. Many times over the 20th century, a promising and seemingly safe drug turned out to have disastrous side effects that were not discovered during its development. In one of the most infamous cases of a side effect discovered too late, the drug thalidomide, which had been prescribed to pregnant women in the early 1960s as an anti-nausea remedy, caused horrible birth defects in the patients' children.

A potentially more dangerous, and certainly more ironic, effect of the success of pharmaceuticals is a rise in the 1990s of viruses and bacteria that are immune to the drugs designed to fight them. Though the effect of drug resistance has always been a factor in drug development, until recently the human race has been able to keep a step ahead in its quest to produce antibiotics and vaccines faster than the pathogens can fight back. The appearance of so-called superbugs may be an indication that, at least in some cases, researchers have reached the limit of what they can do in the laboratory.

Outside the laboratory, however, there are a multitude of plants and other materials in the natural world—the original source of humankind's healing drugs—which may provide the new cures the human race will need.

The following 19 chapters reveal how people discovered and developed the medicinal drugs in use today, describe how many of the most common drugs on the market do their work, show how new drugs are developed, and examine potential threats to human health and potential sources of future pharmaceuticals.

PART 1

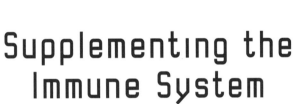

Supplementing the Immune System

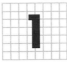

ANCIENT REMEDIES

Many of today's medicines can be traced back thousands of years. Beginning in prehistoric times, people cured or warded off illness using plants, minerals, and even some animal parts that were thought to have natural healing properties. No one can say for sure when or how ancient humans discovered that these materials could make them feel better, whether by noticing sick animals eating certain plants or simply experimenting with different things to see what happened. As far back as 12,000 B.C., though, people living in southwestern France were painting images of what appeared to be shamans, or medicine men, on the walls of ceremonial caves. There is also evidence that people living even farther back in time gathered plants that contained natural painkillers, antibiotics, and other chemicals.

The knowledge of how to use some of these natural healing drugs became mystical lore, passed to a shaman's apprentices along with rituals designed to activate or enhance the medicine's seemingly magical properties. Other treatments were less mystical and soon were part of everyday life. In time, these secrets were written down; clay tablets and other writings from as far back as 2100 B.C. have been discovered bearing recipes for drugs made out of such materials as tree bark, wine, and oil. An even older record provides a better example of medicinal plants in use—the plants themselves, courtesy of an ancient traveler who suffered an unfortunate mishap.

The Iceman's First Aid Kit

It probably was the biggest science story of 1991. Two German tourists hiking in the Alps—a mountain range that crosses the lower portion of central Europe—had come across a frozen body poking through the surface of a glacier near the border of Austria and Italy. At first, local authorities thought the body might be that of an unknown mountaineer from a past decade who had become lost and fallen through a crack in the glacier's surface. Such accidents happened every now and then, and a hiker's body easily could become entombed within tons of ice and not be seen for years.

The truth was something far more intriguing. Teams sent to recover the body discovered that the victim, nicknamed the Iceman, was not like others who had perished in the mountains. When he died, he had been wearing clothes made from hand-stitched skins, a cape made from woven grass, and fur boots stuffed with grass for warmth. He had been carrying tools made of flint and copper, a bow, and a quiver with handmade, flint-tipped arrows. Even his handmade backpack, which had a light wooden frame, obviously was thousands of

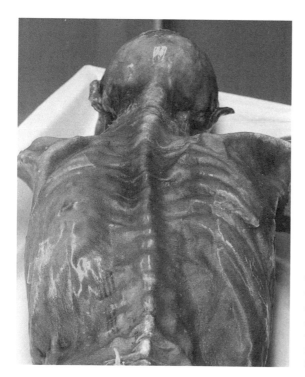

The Iceman, whose body was found in an Alpine glacier, carried a number of possible healing materials. [Courtesy South Tyrol Museum of Archaeology]

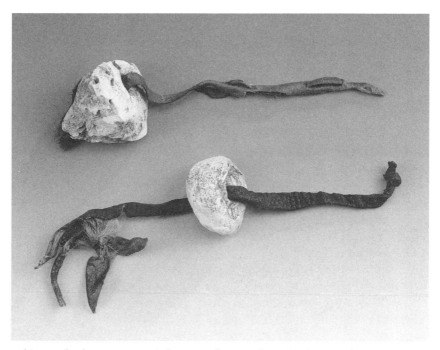

In his pouch, the Iceman carried two mushrooms that scientists now know contain natural antibiotic chemicals. [Courtesy South Tyrol Museum of Archaeology]

years out of date. The ice had been hiding the body far longer than anyone could have expected.

Before long, scientists who were called to the scene, and others who examined the remains in a laboratory, realized that the Iceman had died more than 5,200 years ago and had been preserved, along with the gear he had assembled for his long-ago trek, almost perfectly.

Among the Iceman's possessions were a pair of dried mushrooms on leather thongs. At first, researchers thought they might have been part of the dead man's food supply or tinder for starting a fire. Then a botanist realized the mushrooms were a substance that contained natural antibiotics, chemicals that could kill some types of bacteria or other microbes. The people of the Iceman's day did not know that germs or antibiotics existed, but they could have discovered that eating that type of mushroom could help a sick person feel better. (They undoubtedly also discovered that eating the wrong type of mushroom could kill them.)

Further examination showed that the ancient hiker had been ill before he died: his body showed evidence of repeated infections—the clues were in the fingernails, which showed marks caused by the infections' physical stress—and of an infestation of whipworm, an intestinal parasite. The hiker also had eaten a lot of charcoal, which people use to treat some digestive disorders these days, and had a bark container of charcoal as part of his gear. Together, the mushrooms and the charcoal may represent the first known example of a personal first-aid kit.

If so, it was the first of many such kits to come. When Polynesian explorers traveled across the Pacific Ocean 2,000 years ago and settled on the islands of Hawaii, they took along a selection of trusted medicinal plants. One was the awapuhi-kuahiwi, or wild ginger, which was used to make a soothing cure for stomachache. The plant's thick stems were ground up, mixed with water, and strained to make a clear liquid that was given to the ailing patient. Two millennia later, people around the world do much the same thing when they sip ginger ale to settle an upset stomach (even though most commercial ginger ale contains little, if any, actual ginger).

The most powerful medicines in prehistoric times were within the domain of the shamans, those who were thought to communicate with the gods or spirits that controlled the world, and thus could control disease. It was, and still is, easy for people to believe in a supernatural origin for diseases. Battle wounds, insect bites, broken bones, and similar injuries had causes that were easy to see. Illness seemed to come from nowhere, and thus was seen as evidence of great powers or evil magic at work. An epidemic that hit a village could be punishment from the gods for breaking the laws or taboos of a community; it could be the curse of a witch seeking power or an enemy seeking revenge. According to a Chinese myth, malaria—a serious disease spread by mosquitoes that causes alternating hot and cold flashes—was caused by three demons that enjoyed plaguing humankind. One demon caused pounding headaches with a hammer, a second carried a pail of icy water to chill the victim, and the third had a portable stove that it used to produce a fever.

Believing that diseases had supernatural causes did not prevent people from developing effective treatments, as the Iceman's medical kit seems to show. One of the early emperors of China wrote about a plant whose roots, when ground into a powder, could be used to treat the fevers caused by malaria. This emperor, Shen-nung, also wrote about other herbal remedies in use during his lifetime, many of which still are used today. For thousands of years, the Chinese have used extracts from the leaves of the ginkgo tree to treat coughs, asthma, allergies, and heart and lung diseases. As with other ancient remedies, no one knew why the extracts worked until modern-day scientists were able to isolate their unique chemical compounds. The healing chemical unique to the ginkgo, called ginkgolide B, became known in the 1980s, when chemists at Harvard University analyzed samples of the tree and its extracts. Further experiments with ginkgolide B proved it was the main drug at work in the ancient treatments, because of its ability to relax the muscles surrounding blood vessels and open the lung's airways.

The scientific study of ancient remedies often has yielded practical medicines. Malaria devastated communities throughout Europe and killed explorers in distant lands. After Spanish explorers conquered Peru in the 1530s, though, missionaries to South America were surprised to find that the Inca people had found a simple method for treating the disease. An Augustinian monk living in Peru in 1633 wrote of this surprisingly effective medicine:

> In the district of the city of Loxa *[on the eastern slopes of the Andes mountain range]* grows a certain kind of large tree, which has bark like cinnamon, a little more coarse, and very bitter: which, ground to powder, is given to those who have fever, and with only this remedy, it *[the fever]* leaves them.

The ground bark of the tree, which was known to the Incas as the *quinquina*, became an extremely popular and important medicine in Europe. In the 1820s, nearly 200 years after the *quinquina* bark made its first appearance in the Old World (where it became known as cinchona), two French chemists extracted the bark's active ingredient and named it *quinine*.

Physicians and Poultices

As civilizations developed and flourished, more people got sick. Nothing could stop that from happening: as soon as people started living together in villages, they made it easier for the microbes that cause disease to get around. Fleas had more of an opportunity to feed on people and to transfer the bacteria that cause plague from rats to human hosts. Mosquitoes proved they could carry greater numbers of microbes than just the ones that cause malaria. Worst of all, the diseases that spread from person to person were transmitted with greater speed, and usually with higher death rates, than they had been while people lived nomadic lives.

At the same time, healers who lived in and traveled between these cities shared their knowledge of how to fight disease and, with the development of writing, kept records to pass this knowledge on to future healers. Many of these early medical texts were descriptions of the plants, animal products, and minerals that, alone or combined, supposedly soothed the illness (or at least cast out the demons that caused it). Just as shamans taught their apprentices the magical and spiritual aspects of the healing arts, the medical recipe texts often included rituals to be followed when gathering the ingredients, when preparing the medication, and when giving the medicine to the patient.

The medicines these ancient health-care practitioners compounded were not like the tidy pills, tablets, and capsules that make up most of today's prescription drugs. Some compounds were rolled by hand into pea-sized balls. Many more, though, were powders that had to be mixed with wine or beer. Others were creamlike ointments rubbed into the skin, or poultices that were spread on cloths and applied to sores or other infected areas. Eyewashes, gargles, medicated steam for the lungs—the ancients used these and other methods to deliver the healing power of their concoctions.

In the earliest civilizations, such as those of Mesopotamia (in modern-day Iraq), Egypt, and possibly India and China before 1500 B.C., medicine lay within the realm of religion. Priests were the physicians of their day, and any disease that was not attributed to demonic causes was seen as a consequence of sin or insult to the gods, the dead, or spirits of the natural world. Treating a disease meant purifying the patient's soul as well as alleviating his or her physical problems, and the rituals of preparation were meant to be part of the spiritual realignment.

As the centuries passed, though, the ceremonial aspects of medicine were separated from the physical treatments and became part of the world of magic. Priests began focusing on the spiritual health of the people, interceding with the gods for divine favor, while physicians took care of the needs of the body. At first, physicians made their own medicine, collecting the raw materials at certain times of the year and mixing prescriptions according to special recipes. Well-known healers hired specially trained assistants to gather and mix the prescribed potions, under the careful eye of either the physician or a master of the art of preparing drugs. Eventually, many of the people who prepared drugs set up their own shops and mixed their medicines according to a physician's instructions or by following standard recipes.

The medicine makers' duties combined the work done by modern-day drug companies, drugstore pharmacists, and pharmacy schools. In Egypt, for example, different people collected the plants and other materials for making drugs, mixed the drugs, and stored drugs for later use, occasionally examining them to determine when they should be thrown out. In classical-era Greece (from 600 to 330 B.C.), a spectrum of specialists made up the region's pharmaceutical industry—expert plant collectors, ointment makers, chemists who prepared well-tested remedies, and even drug sellers, who traveled the land selling their wares at markets. Physicians were expected to know how to make their own prescriptions, but many of them relied on the abilities of the professional drug makers.

Ritual did not entirely vanish from the practice of health care, though prayers to various gods of healing gradually replaced magic spells, and many priests had medical and pharmaceutical skills. However, as physicians gained greater knowledge, they realized there was more to illness than a mischievous demon or an enemy's curse. They began to wonder about the reasons for disease.

Health through Harmony

For Greeks and Romans living in the thousand years between 500 B.C. and A.D. 500, balance was the key to good health. Every object

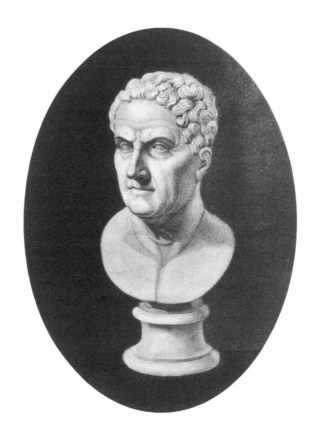

The Roman physician Galen was an unchallenged authority on pharmacy for centuries. [Courtesy of the National Library of Medicine]

in the world, they believed, could be broken down into four substances: earth, air, fire, and water. Trees, for example, contained elements of fire (they could burn), earth (which gave trees their solidity), and water (without which they dried up and perished). These elements were present in the human body as well—or so the philosophers and physicians of the day believed. Rather than possessing these elements in their natural state, the human body had four elemental fluids, or humors, that contained elemental properties. When the humors were in balance, people were in good health; imbalances caused disease.

Blood was considered the humor of air; it was hot and moist, like a breeze blowing in from the sea. Phlegm, which is secreted by mucous membranes in the nose and lungs, was equated with water; it was moist but cold. The other two elements, fire and earth, were represented by substances called yellow bile (hot and dry, like fire), which came from the liver, and black bile (cold and dry, like earth), which came from either the spleen or the kidneys.

Physicians in other cultures came up with similar theories about imbalances in natural forces causing disease. For example, traditional Chinese healing developed around the idea that health depended on bringing the body's yin (the quality found in heat, positive energy, activity) and yang (cold, negative energy, relaxation) into balance. This idea of opposites worked in accord with the interaction of elemental forces within the body, though the Chinese believed in five, rather than four: fire, earth, metal, water, and wood. It was as important to return the body to a state of physical and spiritual harmony as it was to nurse a patient through a fever. The herbal malaria medicine that Shen-nung wrote about represented one way to bring the body back into balance. Acupuncture—piercing the skin with needles at key points to interrupt or redirect the flow of energy through the body—was another method.

The physicians of Greece and Rome classified each drug by how it balanced out the imbalances in the bodily humors. If a patient were feverish—hot and moist—his or her physician might prepare a drug that was made up of cooling, drying elements to counteract these symptoms. On the other hand, the physician might just as easily prescribe a session or two of therapeutic bleeding with scalpels or leeches to reduce the imbalance of hot, moist blood in the patient's body. Other methods that were used to bring the humors back into balance included exercise, special diets, and blistering the skin to draw out the excess.

Three physicians in particular set the course that other medical practitioners in the Western world followed pretty much until the 19th century. Hippocrates, often called the father of modern medicine,

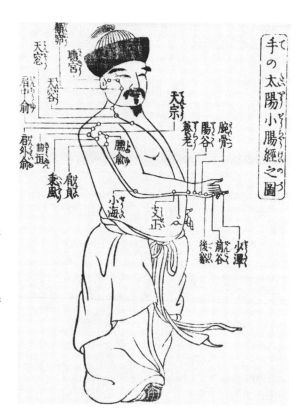

Chinese medical practices focused on bringing the body back into harmony using herbal medicines and other methods. This chart shows a selection of acupuncture points on the human body that could be stimulated to interrupt or guide the body's energy flow.
(Courtesy of the National Library of Medicine)

worked and taught other physicians on the Greek island of Cos around 400 B.C. He and his students were some of the first physicians known to approach their work as a rational and scientific profession, rather than as a matter of magic or religious devotion. Instead of just following the practices of the past, Hippocrates and his students closely watched how their patients responded to various drugs and other treatments, discussed their findings, and experimented with different treatment methods. These physicians were the ones who most actively promoted the theory of imbalances in elemental humors as the cause of disease.

Nearly 600 years later, two other Greek physicians decided to bring a little order to the practice of medicine. The first, Dioscorides, lived in the Roman Empire in the first century A.D. and was an expert on the use of drugs in and beyond the Greek lands. Dioscorides had traveled extensively throughout northern Africa, the Middle East, and the western European land of Gaul (modern-day France), comparing what he knew to the knowledge of physicians who were not trained in the Hippocratic style of healing. At the end of his journeys, he wrote down what he had learned in a lengthy essay called *De Materia Medica*, Latin for "The Materials of Medicine." In this work, Dioscorides described more than 800 plant, mineral, and animal drug sources, along with information on how to use them, where to find them, and even which type of container should be used to store them.

The other physician, Galen, lived in Rome nearly 100 years after Dioscorides completed his work. Galen was known throughout the empire as the greatest physician of his time, and he was a friend to three of Rome's emperors. His great contribution to the development of healing drugs was his system of classifying drugs into three groups—simples, composites, and entities—based upon their effect on the bodily humors. Each drug in the simples group had one of the four elemental properties but no others: heat without moisture or dryness, for example. Composites were mixtures of drugs that combined more than one of the elemental values. Entities were drugs that, regardless of elemental properties, had similar effects, such as causing a patient to vomit (which was a common treatment for many illnesses).

Like Dioscorides, Galen included information on gathering drug-making materials, recipes for different composites, and advice on what types of remedies he found best suited for different ailments. Unlike many other physicians of his time, Galen acted as his own pharmacist and was able to write about drug preparation as a practicing authority on the subject. In fact, his authority extended far beyond his time, and his book *Methodo medendi*, "On the Art of Healing," was published without changes or challenges until the 16th century.

Other physicians in other lands, though, would influence the development of medicine in centuries to come, as would people who were not part of what passed for the world's medical community.

A GARDEN OF SIMPLES

Believing that good health depended on a proper balance of bodily humors was not much better than believing that gods and demons made people sick. The forces that threw the body's elemental fluids out of balance in the first place still were unknown, though the list of suspects included foul air, evening chills, and badly cooked food. At least, the scholars of Greece and Rome were taking a rational approach when they attempted to control amounts of blood, phlegm, and black and yellow bile. There was no way to know that bacteria, viruses, and other microbes existed until after the invention of the microscope in 1590.

Despite the work of these supposedly rational physicians, other healers and educated people still believed in the power of witchcraft medicine. A scholar named Pliny the Elder, who lived during the first century A.D., wrote about a treatment for boils (large, infected pimples) that required a fire and nine grains of barley. The afflicted patient was to take each grain and trace a circle around the boil three times, and then throw the barley into the fire with the left hand. It is difficult to say how this ritual was supposed to rid the patient of the disfiguring malady, but according to Pliny, it promised an immediate cure.

Some other remedies contained truly strange elements, such as brains, internal organs, and even dung from various animals. These ingredients usually were dried and ground into powders that were applied to open sores, burned like incense, or swallowed with beer or wine. Even non-drug treatments could work for or against a patient's recovery. Physicians ordered patients to change their diets and get more exercise as often in Galen's time as they do today, and patients who followed this advice generally became healthier. Physicians who prescribed therapeutic bleeding often weakened their patients enough to kill them.

There were other problems. Well-trained physicians usually worked in large towns and cities. People living in villages far from these population centers were likely to hold old beliefs about what made people sick and how to return them to health. Though medicine men no longer were part of the community, there usually was a farmer or a wise woman nearby who knew how to make simple remedies from local herbs.

Wealth and poverty also determined a person's access to health care. Unless they were new to their art or were generous in spirit, physicians charged a lot of money for their services—and the more famous the physician, the higher the fee he (or, rarely, she) charged. With enough money, poor city dwellers might be able to pay for a compound recommended by an independent drug maker; if not, they had to rely on their own or a neighbor's knowledge of home remedies to pull themselves through their illness.

For most of Europe, life changed for the worse when the city of Rome fell to invading Germanic tribes in the fifth century. In A.D. 395 the Roman Empire, which had experienced centuries of political turmoil and pressure from invaders, split into eastern and western domains. Rome remained the capital of the Western Roman Empire, while the city of Constantinople—built on the site of the ancient city of Byzantium, where modern-day Istanbul, Turkey, stands—became the ruling city of the more powerful Byzantine Empire. Rome was invaded three times in the early fifth century, the last invasion coming in 476. That year marked the end of the Western Empire and the beginning of the Dark Ages of western Europe, when much knowledge, including medical knowledge, was lost or hidden away. People living in the East, however, kept hold of this learning and added new ideas. With time, new medicines and new techniques made their way westward, spurring the development of even more advanced techniques.

Backyard Pharmacies and Old Monks' Cures

With the fall of Rome, people in western Europe were left to fend for themselves. The formerly well-organized Roman territories divided into feudal kingdoms, whose rulers battled each other for greater power and larger domains. People from outside the borders of the old empire invaded these lands in search of loot. The resulting wars combined with the desperate poverty of the common folk to create a breeding ground for such diseases as smallpox, cholera, malaria, and plague, all of which could ravage small towns, large cities, and entire countries with equal ease. Seeking out the expert care of a physician and expanding the state of medical knowledge soon became less important than simply surviving from one day to the next.

Drug-making skills did not die out altogether in western Europe, thanks to the influence of the Christian church. As the Western world sank deeper into ignorance, religious life became one of the few paths open to people who desired a life of scholarship. Priests, monks, and nuns often were the only people in an area who knew how to read and write. Monasteries and convents preserved many of the surviving works of the Greek and Roman physicians; monks in particular copied these medical texts over the centuries to ensure their survival, only rarely adding new information.

More important, convents and monasteries were places where the poor and travelers could find medical care. Members of the religious orders planted medicinal herbs as well as edible crops, and each abbey was sure to have a few holy brothers or sisters who knew how to prepare simples and compounds. The grip of superstition still was strong, however, in the divine seclusion of these religious communities. In the 13th century, one monastery used the following method to treat patients suffering from malaria:

> Take the urine of the patient and mix it with some flour to make a good dough thereof, of which seventy-seven small cakes are made; proceed before sunrise to an anthill and throw the cakes therein. As soon as the insects devour the cakes the fever vanishes.

Of course, in the time it took for the ants to devour the cakes, the patient's immune system would have defeated the disease on its own—unless the disease killed the patient first. Any cured cases of malaria attributed to this recipe were simply the result of luck and good timing.

Outside the religious communities, folk medicine often took the place of formal medical training. Just as modern homes have medicine cabinets full of first-aid supplies, many housewives in the Middle Ages kept a garden of simples, herbs, and other healing plants. These medical crops included comfrey, belladonna, foxglove, garlic, and periwinkle—though some of these, like garlic, were grown as much for their supposed mystical powers (such as turning away vampires) as for their health benefits.

These herbs had been used for centuries, and many of them possessed true healing properties. Comfrey, for example, was used to heal

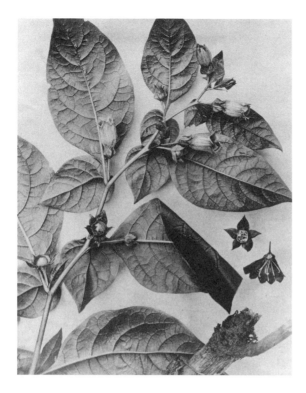

Belladonna, also called deadly nightshade, is a poisonous weed whose sweet berries can kill, even in small amounts. But the plant makes atropine, a drug that dilates the pupils of the eyes, and its juice was used as a cosmetic for centuries. These days, belladonna is used as a source of atropine for medical use and of sedatives such as scopolamine. (Courtesy Eli Lilly and Company)

bruises and broken bones in ancient Greece and in Rome, where it was known as *symphytum*, Latin for "grown together." A poultice of crushed comfrey leaves was tied onto the bruised skin or above the broken bone. This method actually was a good way to speed the repairs to skin and bone; as scientists later discovered, the herb—also known as knitbone, bruisewort, and knitback—contains allantoin, which seeps into the skin and helps body tissues grow. It is used today in ointments to treat skin rashes.

The Apothecary's Art

While the knowledge of medicine stayed essentially unchanged in western Europe, physicians and scholars in the Near East were experimenting with new treatments and adding to the knowledge of their ancient Greek and Roman counterparts. Arab drug makers, who followed new standards of professional pharmacy that ensured the safety, cleanliness, and potency of their medicines, opened the forerunners of the modern drugstore. They also consolidated the practice of making drugs: rather than having separate specialists gather, mix, store, and sell medicines, one person took care of all these tasks.

Arab pharmacists also brought a higher level of science to the practice of making drugs. They used the techniques of alchemy—the science that eventually developed into chemistry—to cook, combine, and otherwise process raw materials into new types of medicine. Rather than relying on theories based on guesswork and philosophy, the pharmacists of the Near and Middle East studied the actual effects of drugs on animals and people, laying the foundation for modern pharmacology.

Some of this knowledge seeped into western Europe toward the end of the first millennium, as merchants and travelers voyaged across the Mediterranean on trading missions and pilgrimages. References to ingredients and compounds that had previously been used only by Arab world physicians began showing up in medical texts copied by the monks of Europe. And when a medical school opened in the Italian port town of Salerno, followed by a school for the translation of foreign texts in Toledo, Spain, some of the first books that were brought in were the works of the Near East healers.

An 11th-century Persian physician and philosopher named Ibn-Sina, whose name was westernized to Avicenna, became one of the world's leading medical scholars. Avicenna wanted to encapsulate the entire body of medical knowledge as it was practiced in his time. Learning all he could about the subject, he wrote a five-volume encyclopedia, which in the West was called the *Canon medicinae* or *Canon of Medicine*. (The word *canon* in this case means a standard, all-encompassing body of knowledge.) Avicenna repeated much of what Galen and Dioscorides had written, but he added insights gained from his own experiences and those of physicians from the Arabian Peninsula to India.

Of the five books in Avicenna's *Canon*, one was devoted to the identification and use of simples, and another covered the preparation of compounds, including an essay on poisons and a list of medicinal recipes. For its time, it offered a detailed description of cutting-edge medicine, and it was used long after throughout the world. When a Latin translation appeared 200 years later, it became one of the main texts used for teaching medicine and pharmacy almost until the 19th century.

By the end of the 11th century, western Europe was emerging from its dark ages and was ready to take part in the world again. Unfortunately for the nations of the eastern Mediterranean, this participation came in the form of 10 crusades to seize the holy lands of Jerusalem, Turkey, and Egypt for the Holy Roman Empire (which included most of central Europe, England, and Italy). The Crusades were not just conflicts rooted in faith, though: the lure of loot, glory, and new lands for Christian kingdoms helped attract warriors to the cause. From 1095 to 1291, European armies marched from their homes to the threshold of the Muslim world, at times succeeding in their quest but ultimately failing to hold onto their victories.

As with all other wars, the Crusades provided a perfect way for germs and parasites to exploit new hosts, and more people perished from disease than were killed in battle. But more than treasure and microbes changed hands. The crusaders brought back the knowledge of Near East scholars, including the advances that had been made in medicine. Some Greek and Roman texts that had been lost returned to the West, and works of Avicenna and others of his time gave European druggists a fresh perspective on their field.

Thanks to the knowledge of the Near Eastern drug makers, the work of their European counterparts moved out of the monastery and

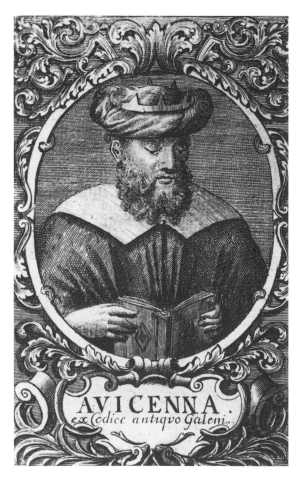

Ibn-Sina, or Avicenna as he became known in Europe, was considered second only to Galen as an expert on medicines and on the proper way to run an apothecary shop. (Courtesy of the National Library of Medicine)

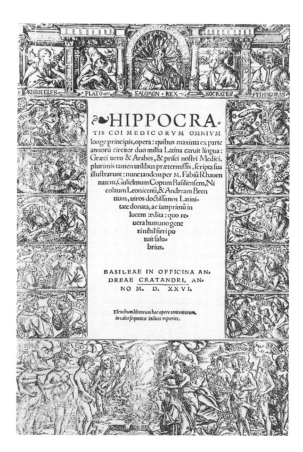

?•HIPPOCRA•
TIS COI MEDICORVM OMNIVM
longe principis, opera: quibus maxima ex parte
annorū circiter duo millia Latina caruit lingua:
Græci uero & Arabes, & prifci noftri Medici,
plurimis tamen utilibus prætermiſſis, fcripta fua
illuftrarunt: nunc tandem per M. Fabiū Rhauen
natem, Guliclmum Copum Bafilienfem, Ni
colaum Leonicenū, & Andream Bren
tium, uiros doctiſſimos Latini-
tate donata, ac iamprimū in
lucem ædita: quo re-
uera humano gene
ri nihil fieri po
tuit falu-
brius.

BASILEAE IN OFFICINA AN-
DREAE CRATANDRI, AN-
NO M. D. XXVI.

Elenchum librorum hoc opere contentorum,
in calce fequentis Indicis reperies.

Apothecaries consulted books such as this one as they studied and practiced their profession. (Courtesy of the National Library of Medicine)

into the streets of medieval cities, where apothecary shops soon became common features of everyday life. The religious orders still maintained pharmacies of their own to treat their members and the poor, but over the next few centuries, their activities were restricted as the professional drug makers gained power in their communities. Pharmacists' guilds began appearing in the 12th century, and pharmacy became recognized as a separate medical profession apart from that of physicians, surgeons, and other practitioners.

Treatments of Dubious Value

For the rest of the Middle Ages, and almost until the end of the 17th century, European apothecaries built and operated their shops according to guidelines that came from the Arab world. Apothecary manuals emphasized the need for cleanliness and order. Ingredients were to be arranged neatly on shelves, scales and other equipment cleaned at least once a day, and old drugs discarded once their potency had expired. Because the apothecary's job was to alleviate suffering and return the sick to full health, the manuals provided moral standards as well, such as charging modest prices and dealing with people in a calm and patient manner.

Many apothecary shops tended to look alike. They were large stalls or small buildings that had a large, open window looking out onto a street or a marketplace. A swing-down shutter served as a counter for the balances, mixing pots, and other equipment used to prepare each day's orders. Inside the shop, rows of shelves held simples and pre-mixed compounds in containers of many sizes and shapes. Customers could watch the apothecary and his assistants at work, much as they could see blacksmiths shoeing horses or weavers dyeing cloth.

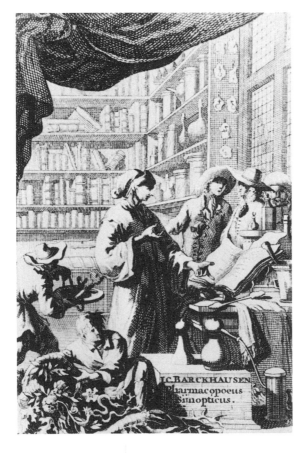

Despite their impressive layouts, the apothecary shops of the 17th century dispensed compounds that often were useless. (Courtesy of the National Library of Medicine)

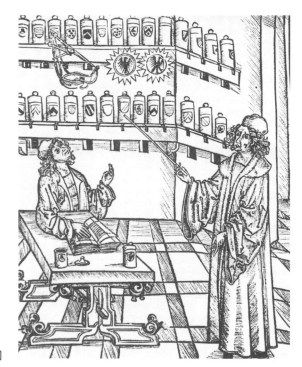

This woodcut depicts an apothecary and his apprentice during the Middle Ages. Most apothecaries learned their profession this way, as formal university training was rare. [Courtesy of the National Library of Medicine]

Later, during the Renaissance period (from the 14th through the 16th centuries), apothecary shops became much larger and more spectacular, with impressively decorated interiors and, in some cases, fully equipped chemical laboratories and nearby herb gardens. Long counters held many of the tools and texts of the apothecary trade, and shelves of ingredients reached from floor to ceiling.

An apothecary in either era stocked thousands of items that made up the *materia medica*—literally, medical matter—of the time. Many of these ingredients had been used for the better part of 2,000 years. Others were new additions made by Arab pharmacists or included by European apothecaries acting on their own information. And, as seen from a modern perspective, many of them were useless.

Three of the oldest drugs, whose origins went back thousands of years, were theriac, terra sigillata, and hiera picra. Theriac was the original "magic bullet" drug: people used it as a universal antidote for poison, an elixir for healing wild animal bites, and an all-purpose medicine for a range of illnesses. Sweet and syrupy, theriac contained up to 70 different ingredients, depending on which recipe pharmacists used, including herbs, honey, opium, snake or lizard meat, and castor oil.

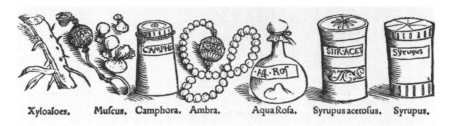

Xyloaloes.   Mufcus. Camphora. Ambra.   Aqua Rofa.   Syrupus acetofus.   Syrupus.

Herbs and other remedies such as these were staples of pharmacology for centuries.
[Courtesy of the National Library of Medicine]

Concocting theriac became a major civic ceremony throughout western Europe, drawing spectators from the entire community who watched their chief pharmacists, physicians, and professors of medicine at work on the cure-all. (Treacle, a modern nonmedicinal mixture of molasses and other syrup, was developed from theriac.)

Terra sigillata had some of the virtues of theriac. It supposedly could treat fever, the intestinal disease dysentery, and plague, and it was taken as an antidote to poison and animal venom. Terra sigillata—its name means "sealed earth"—was a type of clay found on three islands between the coasts of Greece and Turkey. It came from these islands in round tablets that were stamped with seals or emblems showing the island of origin (an early form of pharmaceutical quality control).

Hiera picra, which means "sacred bitters" or "priests' bitters," was apparently a combination of purgative, a medicine designed to expel toxins, and decongestant, a drug that dries up the sinuses and clears fluids from the lungs. A mixture of sweetened herbs and spices, hiera picra was formed into candylike pills for patients to eat. Unlike theriac and terra sigillata, hiera picra was still being compounded and prescribed at the beginning of the 20th century.

Newer additions to the *materia medica* often included magical, rather than strictly medicinal, items. Bezoar stones—masses of hair, vegetable fiber, and other indigestible materials found in the stomachs of animals such as goats—were thought to eliminate poison or other toxins from liquids. Powdered "unicorn" horns—actually rhinoceros horns, deer antlers, or even narwhal tusks—and potions made of precious gems supposedly contained healing powers that could cure ailments ranging from tapeworm infestations to plague.

Then came the "signed" plants, whose shapes or names supposedly were signs of the body parts they could heal. If a plant had leaves that looked like ears, it obviously was meant to restore hearing or cure other ear problems. Lungwort, with its thick, lobe-shaped leaves, was used to relieve breathing problems. Some of these plants provided useful drugs; others had no true healing properties.

The mandrake was the most potent of these signed plants, because its roots often resemble a human body as seen from the neck down. Mandrake roots were used effectively as painkillers, and less effectively as aphrodisiacs, fertility drugs, and good-luck charms. (Scientists later discovered that mandrakes contain chemicals called alkaloids, which can relax muscles.) Harvesting the mandrake was believed to be a dangerous task; a person could die of fright after hearing the plant shriek as it was pulled from the ground. To eliminate this risk, people who collected mandrake tied the plant to a dog's collar and let the dog do the dangerous work.

In general, the state of medicine did not change much until the middle of the 19th century. Even the scholars who charted the anatomy of the human body did not know what made the organs work, what caused the blood to flow, or how exactly a new life came to be. The first medical textbook to be printed using a printing press with moveable type was *De medicina*, or "On Medicine," written by a Roman scholar

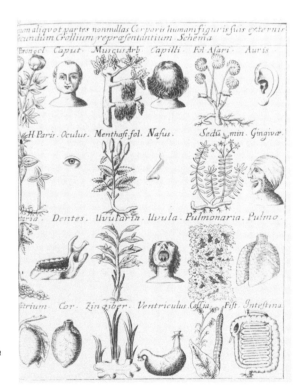

The idea that plants were created to treat the body parts they resembled lasted until well into the 19th century. [Courtesy of the National Library of Medicine]

named Aulus Cornelius Celsus in the first century A.D. but printed in 1478. The book's popularity helped reinforce the ancient theories of disease and their treatment despite challenges from various groups of physicians and pharmacists. These challengers rejected the idea that illness came from imbalances in the four bodily humors. Some of these challengers believed there were no more than three humors at work; others saw their work as the balancing of two chemical properties, such as the level of acids and alkali. It took a lot more work, and a lot more mistakes, before people truly began to understand diseases, drugs, and the human body.

3

PATENT CURES AND MEDICINE SHOWS

The late Dr. Lewis Thomas, a well-known medical writer and president emeritus of New York City's Memorial Sloan-Kettering Cancer Center, once wrote that the history of health care was an "unrelievedly deplorable story." Century after century, he said, "medicine got along by sheer guesswork." Nobody knew why people got sick, and one of the first breakthroughs in medical science was the discovery that some diseases run their course and then stop.

Challenges to the centuries-old wisdom of the ancients were rare, and when they happened they usually ended up creating another set of bad ideas. In the 16th century, a physician and alchemist named Theodore Bombastus von Hohenheim began proclaiming a new way of looking at disease. He said disease was an abnormal chemical condition that disturbed the body chemistry, and it could be cured by strictly chemical means to return the body to its proper chemical balance. Instead of an imbalance of four elemental humors, he said the body was ruled by three chemical principles: the "sulfur" principle of combustibility, or the ability to generate and use energy; the "mercury" principle of liquidity, the ability to move; and the "salt" principle of physical stability.

The physicians who followed the ancient theories of Galen thought that illness could be cured with remedies that opposed the symptoms of disease: if a person had a fever, prescribe a remedy that contained

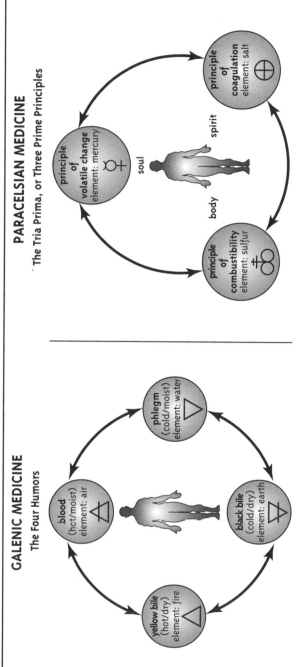

PARACELSIAN MEDICINE
The Tria Prima, or Three Prime Principles

principle of volatile change
element: mercury

principle of coagulation
element: salt

principle of combustibility
element: sulfur

soul
spirit
body

• The body is not ruled by humors but by a series of forces that Paracelsus called "principles."
• Disease comes from *astra*, or motivating spirits, that enter the body and interact with one of the Tria Prima.
• Treatment consists of giving patients medicines that contain the same elemental principles as the one associated with the disease.

GALENIC MEDICINE
The Four Humors

blood (hot/moist) element: air

phlegm (cold/moist) element: water

black bile (cold/dry) element: earth

yellow bile (hot/dry) element: fire

• Each humor has two properties: It is either hot or cold and either moist or dry. The humors also are associated with elements that have similar properties.
• Good health comes when all four humors are in balance. Disease comes from an excess of one of these humors.
• Treatment consists of giving patients herbs or other substances that contain the opposite properties to the excessive humor, although removing the excess (such as through bloodletting) also is an option.

This diagram contrasts the medical principles of Galen and Paracelsus and how they approached the issue of balancing bodily humors.

cooling humors. Von Hohenheim took the opposite position: a patient with a fever needed a drug that enhanced the combustible "sulfur" spirit of body chemistry. He enjoyed the fact that his theory flew in the face of the established medical beliefs. He even began calling himself Paracelsus, a name meaning "higher than Celsus," to show his scorn for the medical textbook written by the Roman scholar Celsus and published 15 years before von Hohenheim was born.

Though his philosophy of disease was little better than that of traditional physicians, Paracelsus had a few positive effects on the development of healing drugs. He and his supporters went farther in bringing the techniques of chemistry to the process of making and analyzing drugs in the West than the works of Avicenna and other Muslim pharmacists did in previous centuries. And the simple act of challenging the accepted philosophies of medicine helped create future generations of physicians who were willing to experiment with new, and frequently successful, methods of treatment.

Such progress came slowly, however, and the field of medicine did not change all that much between 1541, the year Paracelsus died, and the early 1800s.

Medicine Meets Marketing

It was a cold Friday evening in Virginia; December 13, 1799, to be exact. This particular Friday the 13th had been especially unlucky for George Washington, the former first president of the United States, who had picked up a cold. It was nothing much—a sore throat, a fever, and chills—but it was enough to call in Washington's personal physician. Following standard medical practice, the doctor drew a little less than a pint of blood from Washington's arm. The treatment did not work. Washington was still sick the next morning, and two other doctors were called in to assist. They ordered two more "copious bleedings," a hot pack called a "blister" for the patient's throat and feet, and two doses of calomel, a strong medication also known as mercurous chloride.

Washington received another bleeding that afternoon, for a total loss of four pints of blood—two quarts' worth, enough to send anyone's blood pressure to dangerously low levels. His physicians had him force another dose of calomel down his throat, followed by a potion to make him vomit. Finally, "vapours of vinegar," a fine spray of the acidic liquid, were blown down Washington's throat. In all, Washington received the best medical care available in the young United States, easily equal to the treatment he would have received in almost any large European city. Twenty-four hours after Washington felt his first chill, he was dead.

George Washington was 67 years old when he died in 1799. In those days, living to that age was quite an accomplishment, considering that the average lifespan for a man was less than 40 years. But Washington, and many other people then and later, might have had longer lives if doctors had left well enough alone.

In the late 18th century, medicine was more art than science. Doctors relied on "heroic" medicine, which got its name from the large amounts of incredibly powerful medication that physicians inflicted on their patients. The goal of treatment was either to irritate the patient's body into healing itself or to relax the body enough so healing could take place. "Desperate diseases require desperate remedies" seemed to be the battle cry of the medical profession back then.

In America, one of the most influential physicians of Washington's time was Benjamin Rush, who based his techniques on lessons he learned while studying medicine in Scotland. Rush believed that the idea that people were subject to different diseases was nonsense. He taught his students that there was only one disease, "irregular arterial action," and that it had only one cause, "excess excitability of the blood vessel." In other words, high blood pressure made people sick, and bleeding to reduce blood pressure could cure them.

Some medicines also could reduce the "excess excitability." The calomel that Washington's physicians poured down his throat was a purgative, a medicine that supposedly cleaned out the stomach and intestines of toxins that could upset the blood. By purging the body this way, calomel was supposed to relax the body and bring it back into its proper tone. Unfortunately, calomel contained mercury, a heavy metal that the body absorbs easily and almost never excretes. Sometimes, patients ingested so much mercury that their teeth and jaws dissolved under the metal's onslaught—if they were lucky enough to live that long. If not, the metal would concentrate in their kidneys and livers, causing these organs to shut down and subjecting the patients to a painful death. (Mercury was used in rat poison and insecticides until the 1970s, when international law banned their use to reduce the chance of mercury poisoning in human beings.)

As Washington's final day of life shows, patients needed to be heroes simply to live through their doctors' care, much less to recover from their illnesses. "'Tis a very hard matter to bleed a patient to death," Rush and other professors of medicine told their students, and they took this advice to heart. Many patients passed out or died from lack of blood; their weakness, convulsions, and deaths were blamed on the diseases they suffered, not on their treatment.

In some nations, patients bypassed the physician altogether, going directly to apothecary shops or pharmacies for medical advice. For centuries, there had been little difference between physicians, who compounded their own medicine, and pharmacists, who gave medical advice based on their knowledge of treating disease. There also had been little regard for pharmacy as a medical profession. In Britain, apothecary shop owners were members of the Grocer's Company—a professional guild for merchants who sold produce, spices, and other foods—before they formed their own guild to compete openly with physicians. Such arrangements were common throughout Europe in the Middle Ages and the early Renaissance; apothecaries at first were

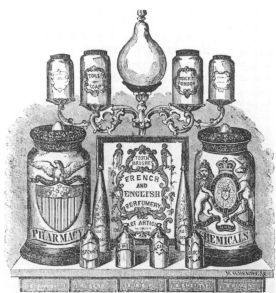

Pharmacy discovered marketing in the 19th century and used it to sell drugs to patients and to sell equipment to pharmacists. (Courtesy of the National Library of Medicine)

TO DRUGGISTS AND PHARMACEUTISTS.
F. HALE,
Member of the Pharmaceutical Society of Great Britain, and of the American Pharmaceutical Association,
46 BEEKMAN STREET, NEW YORK,

Begs to inform Druggists commencing business, or making alterations in their stores, that he has an extensive and well selected stock of Furniture Glass, well stoppered and of superior make, Pine Apple Globes, Show Jars, Porcelain Pots, gold label, Glass Signs, &c., with Drawers, Counters, Show Cases, Bronzed Iron Scroll Brackets, for show bottles, and every requisite for the complete fitting of stores.

From his long experience as Druggist, and general fitter and labeller of stores, he is qualified at once to enter into the wants of his brethren, enabling them to have their stores perfect in every respect, great attention being paid to the dispensing as well as the retail department.

Plans and estimates furnished, with F. H.'s newest designs and improvements.

Instructions for the sale and purchase of business, and valuation of stock and fixtures promptly attended to.   Sep. 1857. 1y called "spicers" because their work, like that of spice merchants, involved grinding plants into powders.

As years went by, strict codes separated the work of the physician from that of the pharmacist on the European continent. In Britain, however, apothecaries fought for and won the right to dispense medical advice as well as prepare remedies, considering that physicians often bought raw materials from a wholesale merchant and mixed their own compounds. Soon, the concept of physician and apothecary merged; the traditional pharmacy functions were taken over by chemist-and-druggist supply houses, which eventually were called simply "the chemists."

Snake Oil Salesmen Hit the Road

With so few options available for medical treatment, all of them equally bad, many people turned to patent medicines. Also called proprietary medicines because their formulas were the property of the companies that made them, patent medicines were pills and potions that had little, if any, real healing power. Though they could be found in many countries, they got their name in England from the royal letters of patent that protected manufacturers from competition in producing and selling a particular product. If he could afford the royal fee, a druggist could entice a king or queen of England to give him a monopoly over an entire class of medicines. Britain outlawed these patents by royal favor in 1624, but the word and the concept both hung on. Patents became legal rights granted to inventors allowing them to make, use, and sell their inventions with no competition for a limited time.

Patent medicines did not have to be safe or effective; they only had to be new inventions. Labels and trademarks were copyrighted, as were the promotional pamphlets wrapped around the product. These medicines, which were called "quack remedies" by those who knew how useless they were, had impressive names like Wizard Oil, Vegetable Compound, Liver Pills, and Backache Plasters. They were put up for sale anywhere their salesmen could set up a display stand and an advertising poster: grocery stores, post offices, barbershops, bookstores, even pharmacies.

The first American patent medicine was a product called Bilious Pills, a "cure" for a variety of diseases, including yellow fever, jaundice, dysentery, dropsy, and worms. The name "Bilious Pills" obviously came from bile, which actually is a chemical secreted by the liver (among other functions, it helps digest fat) but which also refers to two of the humors once thought to regulate the health of the body. Of course, Bilious Pills neither were made from bile nor had anything to do with the health of the liver—the name merely sounded medical and was meant to impress a gullible and uninformed public.

Patent medicines also had something that the remedies of the professional pharmacist usually lacked: a pleasant taste. In addition to bleeding, physicians who practiced heroic medicine relied on foul-tasting medicine to create the conditions for their patients' return to good health. The worse a medicine tasted, the better it worked—at least, that was the theory. Patent medicines, on the other hand, were flavored with roses, sassafras, and other pleasant-tasting plants. For customers who insisted on bad-tasting drugs, some manufacturers dosed their products with herb and root "bitters."

Why did patent medicines sell if they contained no real medication? The fact was that patent medicines *did* make people feel better, but not because they were getting healthier. For most of the 19th century, the two main active ingredients in these fake medicines were alcohol or opium—enough to give patients a false feeling of health while they became addicted to the product. A quack cure called Hofstetter's Bitters, for example, was 32 percent alcohol and 64 percent water, making it a far more potent drink than whiskey. The remaining 4 percent of the mixture was flavoring to make people think the potion was good for them.

Because sales were based on a product's image, rather than on its quality, patent medicine makers created some of the world's first major merchandising campaigns. These marketing efforts pioneered techniques to develop national markets for the product, help merchants sell more of their wares, and use clever advertising in newspapers and on billboards. Legitimate drug manufacturers adopted similar techniques, and some of the most artistic advertisements of the 19th century were for medicines, with images of beautiful women, cuddly infants, plants, birds, and kittens serving to sell genuine and phony remedies alike. Patent medicine companies even ran testimonials from famed writers, actors, and politicians who used their products.

In the 19th century, anyone could advertise almost anything, and they could place those advertisements anywhere the law allowed. There were no national guidelines or ethics for the content of those ads. A small-town newspaper could make sizeable amounts of money from patent medicine advertising, and often such ads were a paper's biggest source of income. Larger papers held to standards that were only slightly higher. Horace

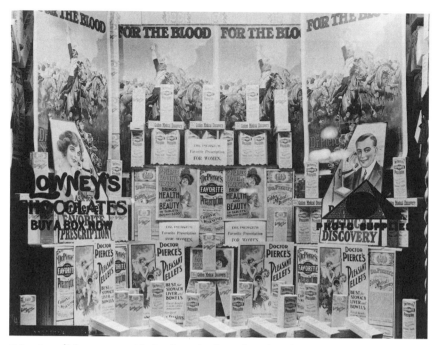

Patent medicines were a big business in the 19th and 20th centuries. No matter how well or poorly such nostrums worked, they could be counted on to draw in loyal customers. (Image courtesy Buffalo and Erie County Historical Society)

Greeley, who founded the *New York Tribune* and was one of the nation's best-known newspaper editors, would not accept ads for venereal (sexually transmitted) disease cures or for abortionists. However, his paper allowed ads for nearly anything else, such as horehound candy that was "good for [curing] spitting of blood and contracting of lungs."

Anyone with a bit of imagination could make a living by mixing some new nostrum and promising a cure. (A nostrum is a medicine made by the person who recommends it.) The self-made druggist had only to mix some powder into pills or bottle some liquid, usually with enough alcohol or opium to make it habit-forming, and then make up a dramatic legend to go with it. One long-selling pseudodrug, Dr. Cunard's Mountain Herb Pills, were packaged with a story of their discovery by the supposed "Dr. Cunard." For decades, the pills' labels told the world about Dr. Cunard's hair-raising rescue of an Aztec princess who rewarded him with her secret formula for the herb pills.

Even legitimate science could be bent to the needs of the patent-medicine con artist. Many people first learned that germs caused disease when they read ads for William Radam's Microbe Killer. Radam was a gardener who decided that killing microbes in the human body was the same as killing bugs on plants. When he began selling his Microbe Killer, which he patented in 1886, he advertised that he could "bring all disease under absolute control" with his "new and Improved Fumigating Compound for Preserving and Purifying Purposes." By 1890 Radam's brochures were attacking medical science, warning potential customers that "to delay for the sake of diagnosis is simply to waste valuable time. It is one of the errors of so-called scientific medicine, and should have nothing to do with the cure." Given the dubious reputation of scientific medicine up to that time, and the desire to save the price of a doctor's visit, people were all too happy to buy Radam's medicine.

Best-Guess Prescriptions

Judge Oliver Wendell Holmes Jr., who later would become an associate justice of the U.S. Supreme Court, called patent medicine makers "toadstool millionaires" because they were greedy and dishonest, and because their businesses could spring up overnight. Other respected

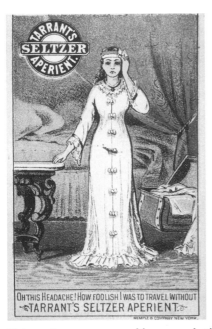
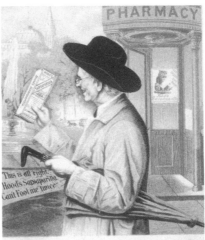

Distressed women, savvy old men, and other characters served to sell headache remedies, sarsaparilla, and other "medicines." [Courtesy of the National Library of Medicine]

figures during the 19th century were equally critical of patent medicines, yet people bought millions of bottles of patent drugs rather than go to doctors.

During the Civil War, patent medicine ads took on a military tone. In one ad, a self-styled "Dr. Judson, Adjutant-General," who seemed to be competing with Dr. Cunard in the mountain herb pill business, issued these "general orders":

> Pursuant to Division and Brigade orders issued by 8,000 Field Officers, "On the Spot," where they are stationed. All Skedadlers, Deserters, Skulkers, and all others—sick, wounded and cripples—who have forsaken the cause of General Health, shall immediately report to one of the aforesaid officers nearest the point where the delinquent may be at the time this order is made known to him, and purchase one box of JUDSON'S MOUNTAIN HERB PILLS.
>
> And pay the regulation price therefor. All who comply with the terms of this order, will receive a free pardon for past offences, and be restored to the Grand Army of General Health.

The ad, which was designed to resemble official notices relating to the Grand Army of the Republic (as the U.S. Army was called back then), was signed "A. Good Health, Lieutenant-General."

Other hucksters of phony remedies did not wait for their customers to "immediately report to" a store that carried their products—they brought the products to their customers. By horseback, horse-drawn wagon, and train, patent medicine salesmen crisscrossed the nation touting the supposed virtues of their "miracle cures." Pausing at every village, crossroads town, and railroad stop, they set up a small stage and started shouting their way through their sales pitch. At first, a well-rehearsed story of adventure, mystery, and romance, focused on the creation of their pills and elixirs, was enough to entice potential customers into parting with their money. As time went on and the nation grew bigger, these showmen expanded their presentations, adding music, juggling acts, acrobats, singers, and even the occasional (and often phony) Indian chief, whose tribes often were claimed as the source of a particular remedy.

Medicine shows and traveling drug sellers were not unique to America or to the 19th century. Wandering apothecaries, whether legitimate pharmacists or con men, have traveled from town to town in every century, visiting small farmhouses and selling their goods in marketplaces wherever they thought they could make a sale. In the era of patent medicine, though, such work was transformed into a grand performance of the art of deception.

Aside from revival meetings, in which traveling preachers delivered impassioned sermons and called on the audience to accept salvation, medicine shows were virtually the only entertaining events that took the time to visit most communities. Boredom and curiosity, rather than a need for a new remedy, often drew people to the performance. Even the most skeptical citizens would show up just to see the show—and go home with a bottle of the miracle cure. There was little fear of being arrested for breaking laws against false advertising, selling untested drugs, or even practicing medicine without a license—such laws did not exist. And where a sheriff or town marshal could have forced a show to leave or arrested the performers, a bribe often cleared away any problems.

Traveling medicine shows lasted until well into the 20th century, and the popular patent medicines left the shelves only when governments restricted or outlawed the drugs they used to hook their customers. Fortunately, while con men were taking advantage of the public's fear and ignorance, scientists were attacking the real causes of disease.

FORMALIZING PHARMACOLOGY

W hile the patent medicine industry was cajoling the public with flashy advertising, legitimate pharmaceutical companies were producing drugs that actually worked. Advertised directly to physicians and pharmacists, "ethical medicines" were sold only on a doctor's prescription, becoming the first mass-produced prescription drugs. They also marked the beginning of a close and controversial relationship between pharmaceutical firms and physicians. As early as the 1820s, drug companies found that, with the correct advertising approach, physicians made good customers. Emphasizing the scientific background of their products not only educated doctors but also encouraged them to write prescriptions for the drugs the companies produced.

At first, these "ethical" drugs were the same ones that apothecaries compounded within their shops; the mechanization of the Industrial Revolution simply made this work faster and yielded more uniform results. Soon, however, large companies began making drugs that were beyond the pharmacist's professional abilities to create. Quinine, the antimalarial drug discovered in cinchona bark, was one such drug. It took a lot of work to separate the drug from the bark, and pharmacists had neither the time nor the equipment to handle the task. Other drugs that required the use of a large chemical factory included digitalis, a heart medicine that was discovered in the fox-

glove plant, and morphine, a painkiller (and narcotic) that was purified from opium poppies.

Existing drugs came under greater scrutiny about this time. For
centuries, large cities produced official lists of approved drugs and
their uses; this type of list was called a pharmacopoeia (pronounced
"far'-ma-ka-pē'-a"). Pharmacopoeias guaranteed that pharmacists
who lived in a city or a region compounded the drugs that physicians
prescribed, but the lists also ensured regional differences. To clear up
these problems, in the late 18th and early 19th centuries many nations
decreed that all pharmacists within their borders would follow a single pharmacopoeia.

Some nations took the opportunity to purge themselves of
pseudomedicinal materials that had been based on superstition instead
of science. Scotland was one of the first countries to drop theriac from
its pharmacopoeia, after a physician published a paper in 1745
denouncing the compound as useless against the poisons it was supposed to counteract. Other nations, though, bowed to tradition and
kept theriac and similar remedies in their drug lists for up to a century
and a half longer.

The first *United States Pharmacopoeia (U.S.P.)*, published in 1820,
took a conservative approach. One section included simples and compounds that the nation's pharmacists were to keep on hand; another
section contained remedies that were part of the traditional materia
medica but were considered (and labeled) as "of doubtful efficacy." It
was up to physicians and pharmacists to decide whether to use the
drug listed in this second section. Later editions of the *U.S.P.*, which
was revised once a decade, gradually eliminated such "doubtful"
medicines.

Classrooms and Battlefields

Along with the new standards for pharmacy, nations set new standards for training apothecaries. Until the late 18th century, the skills
of the pharmacy trade were passed from a pharmacist to his apprentices as frequently as they were presented in a formal university class.
In Prussia (a kingdom whose territory now is part of modern-day
Germany), for example, someone who wanted to enter the profession
in a large city after 1725 had to complete at least 10 years of training
under a licensed pharmacist and complete an academic program at a
Berlin medical college. Pharmacists who wanted to practice in a small
town did not have to attend college; they simply had to serve their

apprenticeship, spend six years or so learning how to run an apothe-cary shop, and pass an examination by a local board of physicians.

France made the pharmacy training process a little more regi-mented shortly after 1800, when it officially established the position of second-class pharmacist. Second-class pharmacists had to meet fewer academic and professional qualifications, but they could only set up shop in rural districts of the nation or in its colonies. Like their Prussian counterparts, pharmacists who wished to work in the big cities of France had to complete a more strenuous course of study and apprenticeship.

By 1820 universities in Europe and the United States were begin-ning to train pharmacists in the methods of what could be considered modern scientific pharmacy. The curricula of these pharmacy pro-grams focused on preparing drugs and dispensing them in proper forms. The pharmacists-in-training also were exposed to the latest concepts of chemistry, botany, hygiene, and other subjects that they needed to know, giving them a good grasp of their field by the time they received their bachelor's degree.

They needed it. The 19th century was a time of great epidemics and wars. Cholera alone killed several million people throughout Rus-sia and Europe in the 1830s. In New York City, thousands died during successive epidemics of cholera, smallpox, and typhoid, scarlet, and yellow fevers from 1866 to 1873; similar diseases swept through cities from Boston to New Orleans. Added to these health crises were con-flicts such as the Crimean War between England, France, and Russia from 1854 to 1856, and the American Civil War, both of which were noted for immense numbers of battle casualties and deaths from infec-tion. Altogether, these epidemics and wars showed the weaknesses of the pharmaceutical industry.

For the United States, the Civil War was the conflict in which more Americans died than in all of the nation's other wars from the Ameri-can Revolution to World War I. Most of those deaths would come not from combat but from disease. Battlefield medicine was mainly a mat-ter of sawing off limbs that were too damaged to save and making the less-wounded soldiers comfortable enough to heal themselves. The more critical medical work took place far behind the lines, in military hospitals and prisoner-of-war camps, which were hotbeds of disease. Malaria in particular found ample supplies of human hosts, while cholera and other diseases also killed soldiers unlucky enough to be captured or simply to get sick. More soldiers died from disease than from all the war's battles combined.

Ether, a painkiller, and quinine, used to treat malaria, were desper-ately needed throughout the war. Doctors in battlefield hospitals on

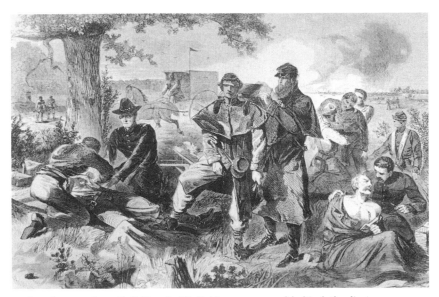

During the American Civil War, battlefield surgeons and behind-the-lines pharmacists contributed to the growing base of scientific medical knowledge. (Courtesy of the National Library of Medicine)

both sides, however, found they could not depend on their medicines to work consistently. One batch might be stronger than another, even batches that came from the same manufacturer. Often, drugs were contaminated either by improper preparation or by poor packaging—neither of which were unusual, considering the conditions of the field pharmacies of the day. Generally, these military drug dispensaries featured a small table and a portable cabinet containing a much-abbreviated supply of standard pharmaceutical materials, sheltered by a tent with one side open to the elements.

Even in the best conditions, field pharmacies only offered drugs that were approved by the national pharmacopoeias of the time. For wartime conditions to improve, there first had to be improvements during peace.

Developing a Targeted Pharmacopoeia

People tend to think of chemotherapy—the use of chemicals specifically designed to treat a particular disease, such as cancer—as a modern technique, yet this is not so. A German bacteriologist, Paul Ehrlich, coined the term in the late 19th century, having built his work on the research of scientists before him. In the 1860s a French physician named Louis Pasteur had announced his germ theory of disease: many, if not most, of humankind's illnesses were caused by microorganisms that infected the body, attacking various organs or emitting toxins that harmed the microbes' host. Scholars in past centuries had suggested that such invaders might be responsible for disease—Anton van Leeuwenhoek, a 17th-century Dutch scientist, found protozoa and other tiny creatures in a drop of lake water using a microscope—but Pasteur proved that infections could be passed under conditions in which microorganisms were the only possible agents.

German bacteriologist Robert Koch, who was intrigued with Pasteur's work, took several big scientific steps when he learned to cultivate bacteria outside a living body. At first, he used cow eyeballs to grow anthrax bacteria. Later, he used blood plasma—the clear, yellowish fluid that remains when red blood cells and other materials are filtered out—to keep the bacteria alive. Finally, he developed a nutrient-rich seaweed gelatin called agar. Each change was prompted by Koch's desire to provide as stable a growth medium as possible, so he could get more bacteria to study in a shorter time. His assistant, Julius Petri, helped speed up the process by making covered, shallow glass dishes to hold the agar and contain the bacteria for easy examination. This innovation worked so well that the dishes have been used in laboratories ever since, and they are now known as petri dishes.

By removing the bacteria from their hosts and observing them under microscopes, Koch was able to follow the entire life cycle of the tiny organisms and figure out how they could be responsible for disease. His first major success came in 1876, when he proved that bacteria caused anthrax, a deadly livestock disease. He followed with similar discoveries for tuberculosis (a lung infection), conjunctivitis (an eye infection also known as pinkeye), and cholera.

With his work, Koch set down four rules for identifying disease-causing bacteria that all other scientists would follow. First, the bacteria must be found in a diseased animal. Second, these bacteria must grow outside the animal's body when given the right conditions to live. Third, the disease being investigated must show up after the bacteria are injected into a healthy animal. Finally, once the disease has developed and a sample of bacteria has been taken from the newly infected animal, those bacteria must be the same kind as those taken from the original diseased animal.

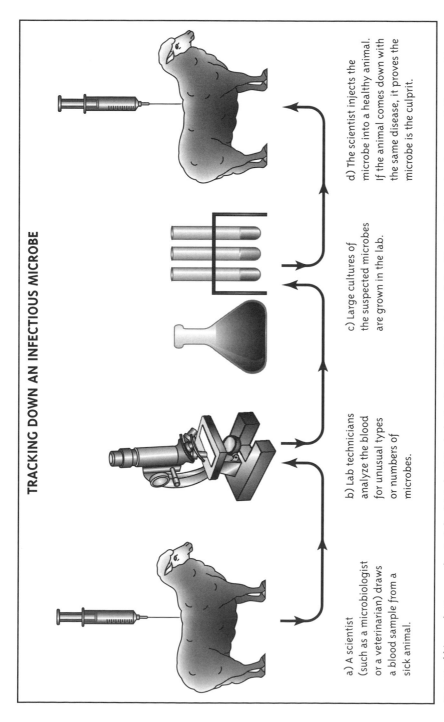

TRACKING DOWN AN INFECTIOUS MICROBE

a) A scientist (such as a microbiologist or a veterinarian) draws a blood sample from a sick animal.

b) Lab technicians analyze the blood for unusual types or numbers of microbes.

c) Large cultures of the suspected microbes are grown in the lab.

d) The scientist injects the microbe into a healthy animal. If the animal comes down with the same disease, it proves the microbe is the culprit.

As part of his work, German bacteriologist Robert Koch devised a method for determining if a particular microbe caused disease. This diagram shows Koch's basic path of reasoning.

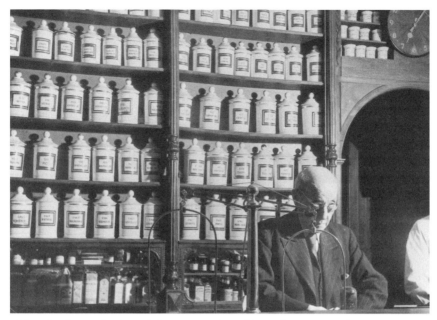

Old-style pharmacies kept their compounds and ingredients out in the open.
[World Health Organization photo, courtesy of the National Library of Medicine]

These findings, and the work of other researchers, put an end to the belief in excited blood, unbalanced humors, and similar semimystical origins of disease. By the end of the 1890s, medical scientists had discovered viruses, mold spores, vitamin deficiencies, hormone imbalances, and other rational explanations for humanity's ailments. Few physicians refused to accept the new ideas of disease transmission, especially after Pasteur conducted a famous experiment in May 1882, during which he controlled the transmission of anthrax among a goat, six cows, and 24 sheep.

There was a major shift away from the heroic therapies. No longer did pharmacists dispense large doses of basic medicines. Instead, they began to fill careful prescriptions for drugs that were aimed at curing specific disorders. Vaccines against anthrax and rabies (both developed by Pasteur), as well as other diseases, began to appear in medical journals and national pharmacopoeias. Some of the assumptions created by heroic medicines remained—even today, people believe that bad-tasting medicines are the most effective—but the overall state of medical practice forever changed for the better.

The mechanics of pill making also were revolutionized. There was nothing new about providing medicine in pill form—ancient pharmacists rolled many of their remedies into little balls, and Avicenna, the 11th-century Persian physician-pharmacist, developed a technique for covering bitter pills in gold or silver leaf. Porcelain pill-rolling tiles, wood-and-copper pill forms, and special pill-forming combs all were standard equipment in pharmacies.

After 1850 machinery began to take over the job of making medicine. Originally hand-operated, these machines stamped out, formed, and coated pills at a faster rate than was humanly possible. Sugar coatings were popular, but gelatin and other edible materials also were used. In addition to pea-shaped pills, drug companies introduced tablets, which were first made using a hand-punch machine developed by an English watchmaker in the 1840s; soft gelatin capsules, developed in France in 1834; hard gelatin capsules, patented in England in 1847; cachets, which were crackerlike wafers that contained drugs; and sterilized, sealed ampoules for injected drugs.

At first, the machine-made, machine-coated pills proved difficult for patients' bodies to absorb. The pills were so tightly packed that they would pass through the body almost in the same shape as they

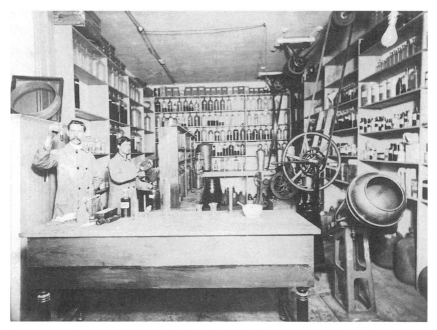

The preparation room of this typical early-1900s pharmacy used the most modern equipment available, including the tumbling machine for rolling pills seen at the far right. [Courtesy of the Buffalo and Erie County Historical Society]

went in, with the medicines unused. Attempts to fix this problem included the use of purified talc and sugar for the coatings, which stomach acids could dissolve easily. By the end of the 19th century, drug companies developed an enteric coating, one that did not dissolve until the pill passed through the stomach and entered the intestines, where more of the drug could be absorbed.

Regulations for the Remedy Makers

Scientists, physicians, and pharmacists continually urged their governments to establish some kind of control over the production and sale of drugs. Part of their goal was to eliminate competition from the unscrupulous patent medicine industry and the traveling drug peddlers who hawked their wares amid circus acts and sing-alongs. Of greater concern, though, was the increasing number of people becoming addicted to the narcotics and alcohol that made up the bulk of these nostrums. It was becoming clear that patent medicines posed a greater risk to public health than did beer or whiskey, the favorite targets of temperance movements.

In the United States, such laws were not passed until the first decade of the 20th century, after a series of articles exposed the hazards to public health that were being marketed by the patent medicine charlatans. Journalists writing for big-city newspapers and for magazines such as *Collier's Weekly* exposed the "miracle cure trusts" the way that other so-called muckrakers exposed the unsanitary conditions of the meatpacking industry and the domination of American commerce by railroad monopolies. The articles described how patent medicines could poison the patients they were meant to heal or get people hooked on alcohol or narcotics.

The Biologics Controls Act of 1902 was the first attempt to regulate the sales of microbes, viruses, and biologically produced medicines such as vaccines in the United States. The law required drug companies to have their plants licensed by the Public Health and Marine Hospital Service. The service's Hygienic Laboratory, which would become the National Institute of Health in 1930, tested each drug's strength and purity. Also, each package of medicine had to be properly labeled and dated, and each company had to agree to "reasonable inspection" of its property at any time.

Regulation of the patent medicine racket, though, had to wait until Congress passed a new law for food and drug companies and ordered the

Department of Agriculture to enforce these standards. Under the Pure Food and Drug Act of 1906, medicine makers were told to redesign their packaging to list how much alcohol, morphine, opium, and other dangerous chemicals were in their remedies. Drug package labels were prohibited from displaying "false and misleading" claims. The new rules also gave inspectors the ability to obtain mail-order patent medicines and test them for arsenic and other dangerous chemicals.

The first case brought by the government under the 1906 law was against Harper's CUFORHEDAKE BRANEFUDE (pronounced "cure-for-headache brain-food"). The company did not tell buyers that its headache cure was mostly alcohol, mixed with some coal tar for color and flavoring. The jury in the case was not asked to decide whether the product was medically effective or safe; the jurors were charged only with deciding whether the label was misleading. Their verdict: the company was guilty, if only for calling its product "brain food."

Of the first 1,000 prosecutions under the Pure Food and Drug Act—BRANEFUDE included—376 were against drugs that made exaggerated claims to cure everything from blood disorders to insomnia; impure drugs; and drugs containing unidentified compounds. Sometimes the government had to be satisfied with small victories. A product called Humbug Oil claimed to cure diphtheria, a throat and lung infection that

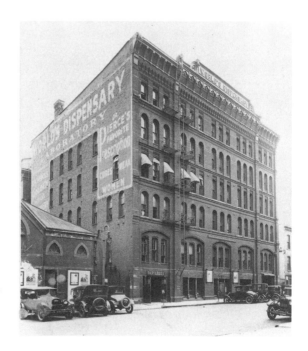

Dr. Pierce's Favorite Prescriptions, which had its "World's Dispensary" in Buffalo, New York, was typical of the patent medicine industry as it existed until well into the 20th century. (Courtesy of the Buffalo and Erie County Historical Society)

can cause fevers, make breathing difficult, and damage heart and nerve tissue. As government prosecutors learned, the "cure" was a mix of codeine (a narcotic cough suppressant), linseed oil (which is used in paints and varnishes), and alcoholic ammonia and turpentine (both of which are poisonous). The company that made Humbug Oil was fined five dollars and forced to take the product off the market.

The most important result of the 1906 act was the reduction of alcohol and narcotics in patent medicines. In general, though, things did not improve greatly. Unscrupulous drug makers still were able to get away with selling useless concoctions as medicine. The authority of the federal government was restricted to a relative handful of violators, such as those who sold their wares through the mail, and courts repeatedly narrowed the definition of what made an advertisement "false and misleading."

It would take Congress two more tries before it passed drug regulations that actually worked: the passage of the Food, Drug, and Cosmetics Act in 1938—following the death of more than 100 people from a particularly fatal elixir—and a series of amendments in 1962. Drug companies now had to prove to the Food and Drug Administration that the drugs were safe and did what their makers claimed.

With basic science research revealing the causes of disease and creating drugs to fight them, medicine was about to enter a new era. A gap remained between professional pharmacists and the drug companies, though. It was as though trained pharmacists wished to avoid the "snake-oil salesman" image that, rightly or wrongly, was associated with all drug makers, legitimate or not.

When the manufacturers became involved in research and began discovering the drugs that they proceeded to manufacture, attitudes changed. The stage was set for some near-miracles in pharmacology.

PART 2

Modern "Materia Medica"

5

A WORLD OF WONDER DRUGS

Joseph Lister was one of the first medical doctors to act on Louis Pasteur's germ theory of disease. He was determined to wipe out the germs whose infections killed patients even after successful operations. This goal was difficult to reach. Back in the middle of the 19th century, preparing for an operation meant taking off one's hat and coat. Surgeons often operated in their street clothes, in operating rooms that also could serve as examination rooms, offices, and personal medical libraries. These surroundings were perfect breeding grounds for microbes.

Given the scope of the problem, Lister's simple methods for combating germs in 1865 were remarkably successful. Lister sprayed the air in his operating room and washed his surgical instruments with a diluted solution of carbolic acid, a harsh, caustic chemical that he thought would be strong enough to kill microbes without endangering his patients. He also required anyone assisting him to wear clean aprons and to put on surgical gloves, or at least wash their hands. Finally, he forbade any surgeon at his hospital from entering an operating room wearing bloody clothes from previous operations or from reusing instruments without sterilizing them. These methods dramatically cut down the number of postoperative deaths in the hospital and brought medicine into the era of antiseptic surgery.

But antiseptic procedures only helped prevent, not combat, infections. Fighting disease meant knowing more about these microscopic enemies, which was difficult. In their natural state, cells are transparent and hard to examine under an optical microscope. In the 1860s, though, biologists discovered that a group of synthetic clothing dyes made out of coal tar were very good for staining cells and making them easier to see. Because a chemical called aniline served as the base of these dyes, they were known as *aniline dyes*. Robert Koch used aniline dyes when he identified the tuberculosis and cholera bacteria, a fact he mentioned during an 1882 medical conference in Berlin, the capital of Germany.

No one could foresee the effect these dyes would have. Certainly not Paul Ehrlich, the pioneering bacteriologist, who attended the conference and became very interested in Koch's methods. Ehrlich had worked with dyes when he was a college student, but had not thought of using them after leaving for work in the real world. When he returned home, he conducted some experiments of his own, one of which involved staining some samples of phlegm from tuberculosis patients. While preparing a batch of slides, Ehrlich worked late into the night, finally leaving his work on the top of a cold iron stove to dry until he returned to his lab the next morning.

Fortunately, Ehrlich did not think to leave a note for his maid asking her not to light the stove. When he walked in that morning, a fire was burning, and the slides, so he thought, were ruined. But when Ehrlich grabbed the warm slides and held them up to the light, he found that they were beautifully stained, with a level of detail that neither he nor any other researcher had seen before. The warmth of the stove had helped the process of staining the samples, particularly the tuberculosis bacteria, which stood out in unmistakable clumps.

Ehrlich applied his technique to other microbes and to samples of animal tissue. He found that an aniline dye called methylene blue stained nerve cells but left other cells alone. This phenomenon gave Ehrlich an idea. As with other forms of aniline dye, methylene blue killed cells. If the dye only attached itself to nerve cells, Ehrlich thought, maybe he could use the dye as a pain reliever, deadening nerve cells without damaging any others. As an experiment, he gave a diluted form of the methylene blue to people who had severe arthritis, and the dye did relieve their pain. Unfortunately, he had to stop the experiment—the dye, he discovered, eventually caused kidney damage.

Ehrlich continued his studies of methylene blue and discovered that the dye also killed *Plasmodium*, a *protozoan* that causes malaria. Better still, he calculated that the amount of dye needed to cure malaria would not be large enough to cause kidney problems. In 1891 Ehrlich gave the dye to two patients who had a mild form of malaria, and they responded immediately to the treatment. This experiment was a major breakthrough. It marked the first time that a synthetic drug killed a specific disease organism in patients during an active infection.

Ehrlich's next target was a protozoan called a *trypanosome* that caused sleeping sickness, a form of encephalitis that made its victims extremely weak and sleepy, eventually sending them into a coma from which they usually never recovered. At the time, the disease—which is spread by a small, biting fly called the tsetse—seemed to threaten half the population of Africa, including the European colonists who had settled throughout the continent. Ehrlich and his assistants tested hundreds of substances, but found none that could kill off the parasite without harming the patient.

In 1906, though, Ehrlich learned from a colleague that the trypanosome he was trying to kill was similar to a type of long, thin, spiral bacteria called *Spirochetes* that, among other diseases, causes syphilis. One of the most persistent sexually transmitted diseases, syphilis causes brain damage and, eventually, death, if left untreated. It had been a devastating, uncontrolled social disease for centuries, as frightening then as AIDS is now. It also was a virtually untreatable disease. Compounds containing the metal mercury were the most effective medicines physicians had to combat syphilis, and those were nearly useless. Not only did mercury have little effect on the spirochetes, but it was toxic to patients.

Ehrlich decided to try attacking the syphilis bacteria with a series of arsenic compounds that he had developed in his work on sleeping sickness. One of his assistants, a Japanese scientist named Sacachiro Hata who joined the lab in 1909, tested the compounds that Ehrlich and his assistants had developed. He achieved success with compound number 606, which killed the spirochete without seeming to harm the lab animals it infected. Tests on human volunteers proved that 606 worked, though not without cost. Arsenic, which formed the heart of the drug, is a potently poisonous metal, and treatments with 606 were painful. Considering the outcome of syphilis, though, most patients willingly suffered through the injections.

Ehrlich named the new drug Salvarsan, a combination of Greek words that meant "saved by arsenic." To make sure that Salvarsan saved rather than killed patients, though, Ehrlich insisted that physicians give the new drug only to their most seriously ill patients and report the results, especially when toxic effects appeared. Ehrlich kept his own record of each dose on charts inscribed inside the doors of his bookcases.

He also insisted on having a sample of each batch of the drug sent to his laboratory so he or his assistants could test it for impurities. After Ehrlich's success with Salvarsan and his pioneering methods for following the use of the drug, every pharmaceutical researcher and laboratory geared up to find other medical "magic bullets." From then on, sick people hoped to be cured with a pill or an injection that would home in on their malady.

Infections in the Trenches

In January 1917, while the world waited to see if the United States would join World War I, the German cargo submarine *Deutschland* pulled up to a dock in New York Harbor. It was carrying a load of Salvarsan for delivery to American pharmaceutical labs for analysis and eventual production. But why would the government of the German Empire transport a load of medicine to a nation that was preparing to go to war against them? In part, the Germans were motivated by common sense. Both the Germans and the Americans knew that syphilis would spread rapidly during wartime—as soldiers on both sides of the conflict met and fraternized with women in Europe and elsewhere—and that the chemotherapy of Salvarsan would be essential. By providing rapid delivery of the Salvarsan shipment, Germany actually was staging a preventative attack—not against the armed forces that the United States would send to Europe, but against the microbes that would take advantage of the conflict to spread themselves among as many victims as possible.

Physicians and generals alike would have been happy to have more drugs like Salvarsan available during the war. Every wound opened soldiers' bodies to invasion by hordes of microbes, causing terrible infections that were almost impossible to cure. The conditions of many military aid stations and hospitals did not help matters, either. Often, the first place a wounded soldier found himself was a bombed-out house or a cluster of tents that had been set up as an initial collection and treatment point. The idea was not to provide long-term treatment, but to patch up the wounded long enough to send them on a cross-country journey to a better facility. Speed, rather than sanitation, was the primary concern, followed by proximity to the battlefield.

Of course, germs did not have to wait for a battle before going to work. The soldiers of World War I, especially those who fought in France, spent most of their time packed in trenches and caves dug into the countryside. Captured soldiers had things even worse, stuck in quickly built (and often poorly constructed) prisoner-of-war camps. These con-

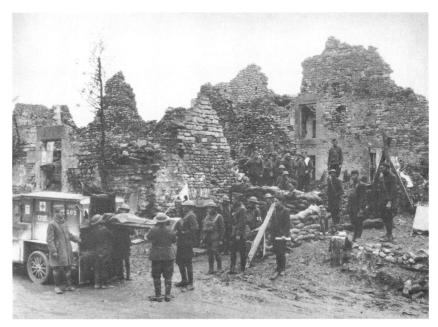

As in all other wars, more soldiers were injured or killed by disease during World War I than were harmed by weaponry. Many of these infections got started in the rough conditions of aid stations such as this one. *(Courtesy of the National Library of Medicine)*

ditions were a perfect breeding ground for disease. By the end of the war, the United States alone lost more than 53,500 soldiers and sailors in battle—and nearly 63,200 to other causes, most of them diseases.

Such death tolls were not unique to World War I. Throughout the history of warfare, more soldiers have died from disease than from weaponry. Soldiers did not even have to be near a battlefield to risk infection. Devastating illnesses drastically cut down the number of troops and almost ended the American Revolution during the encampment of the Continental Army at Valley Forge, Pennsylvania, in 1777 and 1778. A huge number of Union and Confederate soldiers died of cholera and other diseases in prisoner-of-war camps during the American Civil War. And more than 2,000 U.S. troops died of disease, while only 385 died in combat, in the Spanish-American War.

The greatest dangers came from common bacteria that were harmless until they worked their way inside the body. What the world needed, both in wartime and peacetime, was a drug that would cure general bacterial infections. Lister's carbolic acid spray and other precautions were effective in reducing the number of postoperative infections, but working in the stinging mist was difficult, and postoperative infections still claimed the lives of many patients who survived their surgeries. Septicemia, a form of infection also known as *blood poisoning*, could rage through the body after a simple pinprick or scratch carried harmful bacteria into the bloodstream. Puerperal fever, an infection of the lining of the uterus, killed one out of every 500 women after the birth of a baby. Researchers around the world, many of them supported by their nation's governments, spent a huge amount of effort seeking cures for these and other fatal illnesses.

Sulfa Drugs and Penicillin

The German pharmaceutical company I. G. Farbenindustrie established an experimental *pathology* laboratory after World War I to study diseases. In 1927 the company hired Dr. Gerhard Domagk, a biochemist, as director of the new lab and asked him to develop a drug to combat a particularly virulent strain of *Streptococcus* bacteria, the organism that causes blood poisoning. Some chemicals were effective against the bacteria, in particular a gold compound that killed the microbes in infected mice. Unfortunately, these chemicals also were effective against human beings: the gold compound in particular caused serious kidney and liver damage.

After eliminating these chemicals, Domagk turned to a new orange-red dye with the trade name of Prontosil. When the lab's researchers injected the dye into infected mice, the rodents survived. Before Domagk began testing Prontosil on humans, though, he got a call from a physician whose patient, a 10-month-old boy, was dying from staphylococcal blood poisoning. The physician was desperate for anything that might save the baby's life, so desperate that he asked Domagk to send out some of the Prontosil tablets he was testing. This was truly a last-chance effort: as far as Domagk knew, Prontosil only worked against streptococcus bacteria. His lab had not tried it on *Staphylococcus*.

There was no alternative. The physician had to try something to save the baby's life. After four days of treatment, the baby's temperature was down and he was feeling better. Within three weeks, the baby was cured. After this first successful use of Prontosil in a human patient came a more dramatic incident proving Prontosil's power. In October 1935 Leonard Colebrook, a doctor at Queen Charlotte's Maternity Hospital in London, attended a meeting of the Royal Society of Medicine, where Domagk gave a lecture about the drug. Colebrook decided to use Prontosil to combat puerperal fever. In a clinical trial, he treated 26 seriously ill women with the drug, and all of them got well. There was no better evidence that a drug could cure a general bacterial infection.

Still, the reason why the dye killed bacteria was a mystery, especially as the drug killed *Streptococcus* in the body but not in test tubes. Dr. Daniele Bovet, a researcher at France's Pasteur Institute, thought that patients' bodies must be breaking down the dye, separating an active germ-killing ingredient that otherwise would stay locked in the dye. He set out to find this active ingredient and eventually isolated a colorless substance that he named *sulfanilamide*. As a result, Prontosil and similar drugs became known as *sulfa drugs*. Other researchers developed and tested more than 5,000 sulfa drugs, a little more than 15 of which proved to have any real use in fighting bacteria. But during World War II, every first aid kit issued to soldiers contained packets of sulfa powder for use on battlefield wounds. The packets, precursors to the antibiotic ointments of today, probably saved hundreds of thousands of lives. While the war raged, though, researchers already were working on a more effective successor to the sulfa drugs.

In the 1920s Dr. (later Sir) Alexander Fleming was a bacteriologist in the inoculation department of St. Mary's Hospital in London, where he studied diseases and possible means for treating them. One day in 1928, Fleming was cleaning up his lab and sterilizing his equipment, checking each petri dish before throwing away its contents. On one plate, he found large colonies of a yellow mold called *Penicillium notatum* growing over a culture of *Staphylococcus* bacteria. Taking a closer look at the dish, Fleming saw a wide band around the mold, where the bacteria were disappearing. Clearly, something was killing off the staphylococci, and that something appeared to be contained within a yellow liquid that formed at the edge of the mold. Even small, highly diluted amounts of this liquid killed bacteria.

Fleming named this new material *penicillin* and began testing it for any harmful effects. He injected it into a healthy rabbit and a mouse, with no harm to either animal. He mixed it with human blood to see if it would kill off the white cells that serve as the immune system's infection fighters. When penicillin passed that test, Fleming decided to try it out on an actual infection. The chairman of the hospital's inoculation department did not allow his subordinates to test experimental drugs on sick animals. However, one of Fleming's lab assistants had developed a bad eye infection. Fleming had the man wash his eye with a penicillin solution, and the infection cleared up.

On February 13, 1929, Fleming announced his results at a meeting of a professional association called the Medical Research Club. However, no one at the meeting seemed impressed by, or even interested in, the discovery, and Fleming turned back to the research he had been conducting when he discovered the mold on the petri dish. Combined with his director's ban on testing drugs on sick animals, Fleming's disappointment over the presentation almost led to penicillin being ignored. Nearly a decade went by before other scientists began turning his discovery into a powerful antibiotic.

In 1938 Dr. Howard Walter Florey, chief of the Sir William Dunn School of Pathology in Oxford, England, was searching for any natural substance that would kill bacteria without harming other cells. Britain was on the brink of war with Nazi Germany, and Florey knew that keeping British and other Allied troops healthy would be a key to victory. Reading old research papers, Florey came across Fleming's paper and decided to develop a purified form of penicillin. He asked two of his school's researchers to help him with the project: Dr. Ernst Boris Chain, a biochemist who recently had fled from Germany, and Dr. Norman G. Heatley, who was well known for his ability to invent instruments and techniques for working with microscopic organisms.

By March 1940 Florey's team had produced enough pure penicillin to test on and kill germs that cause scarlet fever, pneumonia, diphtheria, and meningitis. They continued purifying penicillin and soon had enough to test the drug on mice that were infected with *Streptococcus*. The new drug killed bacteria in living animals without injuring their hosts. The first human treated with the drug, a 43-year-old Oxford police officer named Albert Alexander who had developed a serious

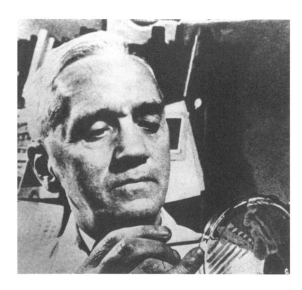

Sir Alexander Fleming discovered penicillin and its ability to destroy bacteria while analyzing the mold *Penicillium notatum* in 1928.
(Courtesy of the National Library of Medicine)

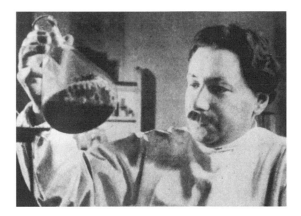

Dr. Ernst Boris Chain was a 29-year-old biochemist when he joined the team that refined penicillin. (Courtesy of the National Library of Medicine)

infection after scratching himself on a rose thorn, improved rapidly until the team ran out of their extremely limited supply of the drug. Later, though, a 14-year-old boy and a six-month-old baby survived after treatments, and people began describing penicillin as a "miracle drug."

Antibiotics from the Jet Age to the Millennium

Penicillin proved itself just in time to save millions of lives during World War II. For the first time in its history, military deaths from infections were fewer than the number of deaths in combat. Penicillin also sparked a worldwide hunt for similar drugs: No one knew how many thousands of different molds and fungi might become medicines. The Bristol-Meyers Company in Syracuse, New York, sent envelopes to its stockholders, asking them to send soil samples from their cellars, gardens, and yards. Other pharmaceutical companies asked for mold samples from missionaries, foreign correspondents, pilots, prospectors, and anyone else who traveled around the world.

Dr. Selman Waksman, a professor at Rutgers University in New Jersey and a researcher for pharmaceutical manufacturer Merck and Company, coined the word *antibiotic* in 1942 to describe chemicals that interfere with the life of a microorganism. He discovered a powerful antibiotic, streptomycin, when he tested a mold that one of his students found in a chicken's throat. Amazingly, the drug killed tuberculosis bacteria—physicians had hoped penicillin would wipe out tuberculosis, but it had not—as well as some kinds of pneumonia and other infectious microbes. Waksman also was a humanitarian pioneer. Ordinarily, the company that discovers a new drug has exclusive rights to produce and sell that drug. Waksman, however, believed that streptomycin was too important to be limited to one drug company and convinced Merck to give up its exclusive rights so that other companies could produce streptomycin.

The 1940s were a period of explosive growth in antibiotics, whose effects were so remarkable that people began referring to them as wonder drugs. Fungus in a soil sample from Venezuela yielded the drug chloromycetin, a *broad-spectrum* antibiotic that killed many bacteria, including the *Rickettsia* bacteria that causes Rocky Mountain spotted fever and typhus. A sample of loam (soil) from Missouri contained a fungus that produced Aureomycin, which not only was a broad-spectrum antibiotic but also destroyed some large viruses, making it the world's first antiviral drug. In 1949 researchers at Pfizer found a remarkable antibiotic in soil sample from a backyard near the company's Terre Haute, Indiana, headquarters. At the time, penicillin fought 25 different diseases, and streptomycin was effective against 15 organisms. The new antibiotic, Terramycin, could combat 100 different diseases, including scarlet fever and pneumonia. Pfizer began producing Terramycin only a few months after its discovery.

Antibiotics usually get their names from the organisms that originally produced them. Terramycin came from the previously unknown fungus that was named after Terre Haute. Miamycin came from a fungus found in Miami, Florida, and Nystatin came from the New York State Board of Health laboratory, where it was identified. Sometimes scientists do not stick to place-names. The scientists who discovered

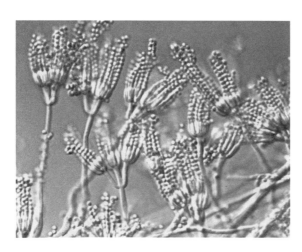

The mold *Penicillium notatum* yielded the world's first modern antibiotic. [Jim Deacon, University of Edinburgh]

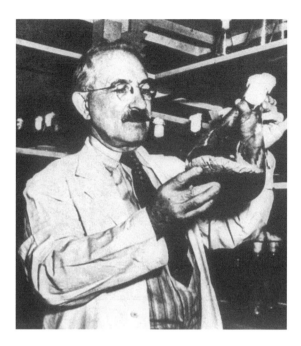

Dr. Selman Waksman coined the word *antibiotic* in 1942. He also discovered the drug streptomycin, which was an effective treatment against tuberculosis.
[Courtesy of the National Library of Medicine]

Doricin and Helenin named them after their wives, and Seramycin was named after a mother-in-law.

The increase in travel created by jet airplanes and interstate highways both helped and hampered the search for new antibiotics starting in the 1950s. It helped by making it easier for drug hunters to get samples of fungi and other sources of potentially life-saving drugs. It hampered by making it easier for disease microbes to spread themselves, share genes, and become resistant to the drugs already in use. (Chapter 16 discusses drug resistance more fully.) Still, antibiotics were so amazingly effective, and amazingly profitable, that drug companies spurred on the search for more powerful products. Things became a little easier in 1957, when researchers developed a way to synthetically produce penicillin, creating the chemical without having to harvest it from either *Penicillium* or *Aspergillis*, another mold that also turned out to produce the drug. From then on to the present day, drug makers have been able to produce larger quantities of some antibiotics even as they discover new ones.

PREEMPTIVE STRIKES

Modern drugs can cut down the time people suffer from illness and injury, and even can prevent germs from gaining a foothold in the body in the first place. Drugs such as vaccines and anesthetics are the result of centuries of work that started in the 18th century, when physicians began examining old-time folk remedies and healing techniques. These traditional remedies became the starting point of research into creating reliable and easy-to-control drugs that have formed much of the modern chemical arsenal against disease and pain.

Two of the most important of these discoveries was the concept of *inoculation*, preparing the immune system to fight a disease by introducing it to small amounts of the disease's microbes, and the creation and refinement of *anesthetics*, drugs that patients receive before surgery. Though they have different purposes, both types of drugs interrupt processes that keep the body from maintaining its health. And, as with other aspects of medicine, both have roots that stretch well back into history.

Seeking Paths around Illness and Pain

People were warding off disease chemically long before the days of Pasteur and Koch. In ancient Egypt, the armies of laborers who built the pyramids had ample supplies of onions, garlic, and similar foods in their diet. Modern scientists have discovered that these edible bulbs and herbs contain natural antibiotics. Some experts on ancient Egyptian life believe that these foods may have served as a form of preventative medicine as much as a source of nutrition. Though the Egyptians did not know about microbes, they may have noticed that people who ate plenty of these foods were healthier than those who did not.

Much ancient health care involved acting on these types of observations. People around the world were well aware that certain conditions—the change of seasons, floods, famine, war, and similar events—coincided with the rise or spread of disease. Some civilizations found remarkably practical solutions to these problems, such as draining swamps to eliminate the "bad air" that supposedly caused illnesses. In the process, of course, this work would cut down the number of insects that spread such diseases as malaria. In other times, people tried more desperate measures to interrupt what they thought was the path of transmission. During the great epidemic of bubonic plague that struck Europe in the 14th century, people in some areas thought that cats were causing the disease, and responded by killing and burning every cat they could catch. In reality, the cats had been busy catching rats that carried the fleas that were spreading the plague bacteria. Residents of affected areas could not make that connection, though. All they could see was a lot of cats near where people were dying of the plague, and they acted on this observation.

Fortunately, people began responding a little more rationally as they learned more about diseases. Physicians gradually learned how to track diseases to their source and use this knowledge to prevent further cases, a practice that formed the basis of *epidemiology*. A classic story of how this field developed involves a London doctor, John Snow, who was personal physician to Queen Victoria in 1849, during a serious cholera outbreak. Snow and other physicians noticed that a large number of cholera victims lived in one neighborhood, where 500 people came down with the disease in less than two weeks. Snow decided to investigate, and after talking with the victims he discovered that all the patients drank and washed with water from a single public water pump. When London officials, acting on his advice, disabled the pump by removing its handle, the number of new cholera cases in the area dropped remarkably.

It would have been nice if simple measures like Snow's were available for all epidemics, but the fact is that disease microbes can travel along a nearly unlimited number of paths into the body. They can enter through the nose or mouth, lodging in the nasal cavity, the throat, the lungs, or the stomach. They can ride in through an insect bite. They can land on the skin and start growing in the pores. They even can spend years lurking in the body, becoming active only when the immune system is fighting another illness. Attacking the microbes themselves is almost the only way to fight them.

Compared to the effort it takes to kill microbes, killing pain is easy. For thousands of years, farmers in India, Africa, China, Asia Minor, and Mexico gathered dried juice from the unripe seedpods of *Papaver somniferum*, the white poppy, and used it as the main ingredient of powerful, pain-reducing drugs. The Greeks called this juice *opion*, and used it to make a *narcotic* (sleep-inducing) drug called *opium*. Opium also served as a medicine against the pain of injury or infection. One second-century-B.C. toothache remedy called for a mixture of opium, black pepper, saffron, and the seeds of anise, carrots, and parsley.

Opium continued as part of the world's *materia medica* for thousands of years. Thomas Sydenham, an English physician in the 1660s, wrote of opium that "there is not one that is equal in its power to moderate violence of so many maladies and even to cure some of them." He mixed opium with saffron and wine to make a drug he called *laudanum*, which physicians relied on until the early 20th century. Other scientists analyzed opium to discover the secrets of its miraculous abilities in hopes of finding a safer painkiller. In 1803 Frederick Sertürner extracted pure, odorless, and bitter crystals from the raw opium poppy juice and named the substance *morphine*, for Morpheus, the Greek god of dreams. It was a powerful drug, capable of relieving severe pain without causing unconsciousness and without interfering with any of the senses. It also was a dangerous drug. After he tested morphine on dogs, Sertürner tested the drug on himself, and almost died from an overdose. He later used smaller doses of the drug to prove that it was safe for human use.

From basic starting points such as these—the attempts to stop disease through diet and detective work, the refinement of ancient herbal drugs into potent painkillers—scientists developed two categories of drugs that worked by short-circuiting the pathways of illness and pain.

Vaccination

Part of the immune response involves creating *antibodies* to microbes that make their way into the body. Antibodies are protein molecules that attach themselves to the surface of *antigens*, the foreign microbes that invade the body. In a way, each antibody acts like a self-guided missile, seeking out and destroying a particular type of bacterium or virus. Each time the immune system encounters and defeats a new antigen, it produces a new type of antibody designed to attack that particular threat. The more diseases a person survives, the greater his or her arsenal of antibodies, and the greater the chance of warding off future infections.

Sometimes, though, a disease is so powerful that only a small number of people survive to develop antibodies. Smallpox—a potentially fatal disease that can cover the body with tiny, pusfilled bumps—has been all but eradicated, but for centuries, it was one of the world's most feared diseases. Nearly every family had at least one member who died from the pox. Even so, in every town stricken with smallpox there were a fortunate few who either never came down with the disease or developed a mild case and survived (though they were marked for life with pit-shaped scars). As far back as the 11th century, healers in China and western Asia noticed that the people who survived an attack of smallpox seldom got the disease again. Though the physicians did not know the reasons behind this phenomenon, they learned to turn it to their advantage, and for centuries many people living east of the Mediterranean Sea did not fear smallpox quite as much.

Lady Mary Wortley Montagu, the wife of England's ambassador to Turkey in 1716, saw the reason for this lack of fear firsthand. Old women would go from house to house in Istanbul, the city where Lady Mary lived, carrying nutshells filled with pus taken from people who had mild cases of smallpox. They would scratch the arm of each person in the house who

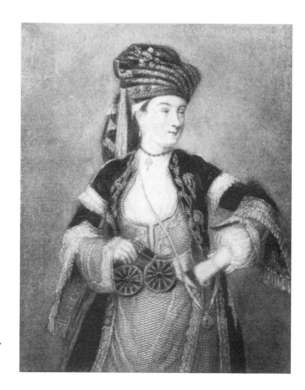

Lady Mary Wortley Montagu discovered the "heathen" practice of smallpox inoculation while in Turkey in 1716. When she returned to England, she persuaded King George I to have his grandchildren inoculated.
[Courtesy of the National Library of Medicine]

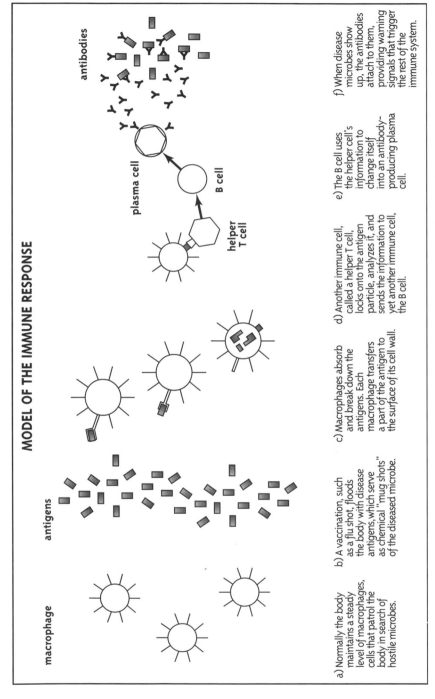

MODEL OF THE IMMUNE RESPONSE

macrophage

antigens

plasma cell

B cell

helper
T cell

antibodies

a) Normally the body maintains a steady level of macrophages, cells that patrol the body in search of hostile microbes.

b) A vaccination, such as a flu shot, floods the body with disease antigens, which serve as chemical "mug shots" of the diseased microbe.

c) Macrophages absorb and break down the antigens. Each macrophage transfers a part of the antigen to the surface of its cell wall.

d) Another immune cell, called a helper T cell, locks onto the antigen particle, analyzes it, and sends the information to yet another immune cell, the B cell.

e) The B cell uses the helper cell's information to change itself into an antibody–producing plasma cell.

f) When disease microbes show up, the antibodies attach to them, providing warning signals that trigger the rest of the immune system.

Vaccinations provide a generally safe means of warning the immune system about serious infections that it may come across.

had not yet had the disease, smear a bit of the infected fluid in the cut, and tie a nutshell over the site. About a week later, the treated people would come down with mild symptoms of smallpox and recover a few days later. From then on, they almost never came down with the disease.

Lady Mary had her three-year-old son receive the procedure and tried to convince physicians she knew to adopt the procedure when she returned to England. Eventually, she persuaded authorities at London's Newgate Prison to inoculate six prisoners, who were promised pardons for volunteering, and convinced King George I to have his two grandchildren inoculated. However, the procedure was too risky to apply it to the public at large. The infection could suddenly get out of hand, creating a serious case of the disease rather than the mild effect people desired. The world needed a safer method.

Dr. Edward Jenner found it. A physician, Jenner knew of a popular belief that connected milking cows to immunity from smallpox. Farmers and milkmaids sometimes got a disease called *cowpox* from their dairy herds that caused sores on the milker's skin. These sores eventually healed, but the mild malady seemed to make its victims immune against smallpox. In 1796 Jenner decided to put this phenomenon to a scientific

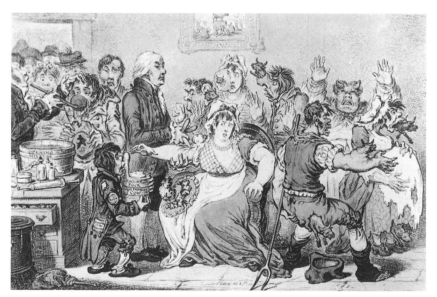

Edward Jenner's cowpox "ingrafting" experiment was greeted with as much ridicule as respect. The antivaccination society that published this cartoon showed Jenner's patients growing cows, or growing into cows, after their inoculation. [Courtesy of the National Library of Medicine]

test. He took some pus from the hands of a milkmaid and scratched it into the skin of an eight-year-old schoolboy. After the boy's cowpox sores healed, Jenner repeated the procedure with a sample of smallpox pus. The boy did not develop even a mild case of the more serious disease.

Jenner published the results of his work in 1798. He called his procedure *vaccination*—naming it with the Latin word for cow, *vacca*—and referred to cowpox as *variolae vaccinae*—*variolae* coming from the Latin word for smallpox and *vaccinae* indicating that this particular form of pox came from cows. Jenner had no idea what caused smallpox, nor did he have any idea how vaccination worked. For the first time in history, though, people could choose to be vaccinated and become immune to the deadly or disfiguring disease. Many chose not to, either because the procedure still had risks or because they simply did not understand the process. (A political cartoon of the time poked fun at vaccination, showing people who received it growing tiny cows from just about every part of their bodies.)

Jenner's work contributed to the development of modern immunology, even though 100 years would pass before anyone found out about the immune system and how it works. Until that time, physicians and other medical scientists were able to create vaccines against other diseases simply by analyzing their effects and, at times, their microbes. In most cases, they were able to kill or weaken germs with chemicals or heat, or use naturally mild-acting microbes, to introduce the body's defenses to the disease. They did not even have to identify the microbe to fight it. In 1885 Louis Pasteur discovered a vaccine that prevented rabies, a disease that was then always fatal. Today, we know that rabies comes from a virus, but Pasteur did not know the cause of rabies, except that he knew it came from a germ that was too small to appear in his microscope. The rabies vaccine was unusual, as it had to be administered *after* a patient already had been exposed to the disease (usually through an animal bite). If the weakened germ reached the immune system in time, though, it could "kick start" the body's production of antibodies, effectively warning the body that the disease was already present.

As scientists learned more about disease microbes, more vaccines appeared. Vaccines against tetanus, diphtheria (an often-fatal respiratory system disease), and a host of other illnesses saved countless lives. In the process, these medicines changed the way people lived. *Poliomyelitis*, or polio, terrified everyone in the United States and Canada between the 1920s and the 1940s. The virus that causes the disease attacks and inflames the gray matter in the spinal cord; in fact, *polio* and *myel* come from the Greek words for gray and marrow. (The suffix *itis* means "disease of.") In its most serious forms, polio causes partial or total paralysis; because polio's most frequent victims are very young children, people also call it *infantile paralysis*. In the late 1930s, an organization called the National Foundation for Infantile Paralysis (later called the March of Dimes Birth Defects Foundation) began a nationwide fund-raising and research drive to find either a vaccine against or a cure for the disease.

It took nearly a decade and a half for the work to pay off. Dr. Jonas Salk, a microbiologist who helped establish the foundation, developed a vaccine in 1952 using viruses that he killed with a solution of formaldehyde. The structures of the dead viruses were intact, giving the immune system the pattern it needed to create antibodies of the proper shape. The vaccine went through a series of mandatory government tests and reviews over the next two years, and in April 1954 a selection of elementary school students across the nation lined up for the world's first polio vaccinations. The results were wildly successful. There are three types of poliovirus, and Salk's vaccine effectively prepared the students' immune systems to combat all three. The only problems with the vaccination came a year later, when 250 children came down with and died from the disease after being inoculated. An investigation revealed that 150 of these deaths came from a batch of vaccine in which the viruses had not been killed; the rest were students who already had started developing polio or who simply did not build up immunity.

Interestingly, Salk's dead-virus vaccine would be succeeded by one that used live poliovirus. Dr. Albert Sabin, a Russian-born American physician and microbiologist, had been working with live polio viruses since the mid-1930s and was convinced that making a safe vaccine from live, but weakened, polio viruses was possible. And it would be cheaper and easier to give because it would not have to be injected: It could be eaten. By 1957 Sabin had a vaccine made from the three kinds of live polioviruses, and over the next two years gave it in sweet syrup or candy to children in Russia, Poland, Mexico, and Singapore. He had to go outside the United States to test it because most American children had been given Salk's vaccine by then. Fifteen million children received Sabin's vaccine, with very few ill effects. In 1960 the United States government approved the oral vaccine, which was given out in sugar cubes rather than hypodermic needles.

These vaccines and the many others that have been developed are some of the best of all drugs because they stop diseases before they start, and because they save millions of dollars in health care that can be spent on other maladies. They are so effective that in 1980, when United Nations health officials found that only 20 percent of the world's children had been vaccinated against the big killer diseases, they started a major worldwide vaccination campaign. By the 1990s, 80 percent of all children in the world under age one had been immunized, more than likely saving millions of lives.

Anesthesia

Morphine was the first chemically active ingredient extracted from a plant, and its discovery was a huge step forward in the history of pharmaceuticals. Once drug manufacturers know the active ingredient of a crude drug, they can design more accurate doses, getting rid of impurities and controlling any toxic effects. Even better, as chemists began working out the exact chemical structure of a drug's active ingredient, they figured out ways to synthesize it from other chemicals, such as coal tar.

Morphine also was one of the first chemicals extracted specifically as an anesthetic. There were others, though. In 1799 an English chemist named Humphrey Davy developed nitrous oxide, a colorless, odorless gas. Davy had no idea what the gas could be used for, as no one had encountered it before: It was the end result of Davy's pioneering research into gaseous substances. To see what effects the gas might have, Davy produced and inhaled about 16 quarts of it. He later wrote that it eliminated all sense of pain and made him feel "absolutely intoxicated." This second effect caused people to laugh giddily and gave nitrous oxide its common name, "laughing gas," and while Davy and other scientists investigated using nitrous oxide as a painkiller during surgery, the gas also became the central attraction of parties called "laughing gas frolics." The first known use of nitrous oxide as a medical anesthetic came in 1844, when a Boston dentist named Horace Wells used it while he extracted one of his own teeth, which had become badly infected. (Physicians and chemists often tested new drugs or methods on themselves before using them on patients.)

Though effective, nitrous oxide only had a mild effect on patients, dulling pain enough for dental procedures but not enough for critical operations. What surgeons needed was an anesthetic that was strong enough to numb pain throughout the entire body—a general anesthetic. A physician in Jefferson, Georgia, named Crawford Long found such a painkiller in 1842, when he staged a "laughing gas frolic" using sulfuric ether rather than nitrous oxide. After noticing that some of his friends were bruised but had felt no pain, he used the gas on a patient who needed a cyst removed. Another Boston dentist, William Morton, discovered ether on his own in 1846 (Long did not publish the results of his work until 1849). Morton used the gas to anesthetize a patient who needed a tooth pulled. Morton's patient went to a local newspaper with the story of Morton's "painless dentistry," and a Boston surgeon convinced Morton to demonstrate his technique at the city's Massachusetts General Hospital. There, a surgeon used Morton's procedure to anaesthetize a patient who needed to have a mild tumor removed. After Morton, Long, and other physicians began publicizing the benefits of ether, it became a standard feature of surgical operations. A third anesthetic, chloroform, came into being in 1831, when two chemists— one in the United States, one in Germany—invented it independently.

These three chemicals marked the start of modern anesthesia, but more was needed to make it easier for patients to bear the rigors of surgery. General anesthesia can be dangerous: giving patients a little too much will relax their bodies to the point where they shut down. Surgeons needed a way to numb just the part of the body that needed surgery. In 1884 they got it. Two surgeons in New York City, William Halsted and an ophthalmologist named Carl Killer, used small amounts of cocaine either injected into a patient's body or applied with drops to a patient's eye. Known today mainly as an addictive street drug, cocaine comes from the South American coca plant; people living in and around the Andes have used its leaves as an energy booster and painkiller for centuries. Chemists separated cocaine from the leaves of the coca plant in 1859 and had demonstrated its ability to deaden pain, but physicians mostly ignored it until Halsted and Killer adopted it in their own practices.

Part of the reason for the delay was a lack of an effective way to deliver the drug. For a drug to work, it has to reach the bloodstream; the more rapidly it reaches the bloodstream, the faster it works. Taking pills, potions, or other compounds by mouth is an easy way to get medicine into the body, but it takes a while for the stomach and intestines to break down and absorb the drug. For millennia, physicians used needles, hollow reeds, and even small cuts in the skin to speed up this process. It was 1853, though, before doctors had access to a practical *hypodermic* ("beneath the skin") syringe. Invented by Dr. Alexander Wood, an American physician, it looked very much like its modern descendant: a hollow needle attached to a thin glass cylinder, with an airtight and watertight piston to drive drugs into the body.

The invention of the hypodermic syringe expanded the options available to drug makers and physicians in administering drugs. For anesthetics in particular, syringes gave physicians the ability to place painkillers exactly where they needed to go, without having to expose the entire body to unneeded, and possibly dangerous, amounts of chemicals. It also provided the means for an unexpected, and unwanted, side effect: addiction to these potent chemicals, which captured many of the physicians who pioneered their medical uses. Still, by the turn of the century, the beneficial effects of these chemicals established anesthesiology as a revolutionary presence in the medical world.

7

BIOLOGICAL SYSTEMS MANAGEMENT

Vaccines, anesthetics, antibiotics—people are accustomed to taking these and other chemicals into their bodies for their health. Of greater importance, though, are the chemicals that naturally exist in the body. Humans are walking chemical factories whose lives largely are determined by the compounds that their cells produce every second of their lives. Blood, of course, is a rich chemical "soup," a broth of plasma that transports red cells, platelets, nutrients, antibodies, and other substances. Lying alongside the blood vessels is the *lymphatic system*, a separate pipeline that carries white blood cells to infected areas, removes bacteria, and carries fat from the small intestine to the rest of the body.

Then there is the *endocrine system*, a series of glands that constantly adjusts the body's metabolism, keeping the internal environment stable in response to changes in activity, temperature, nutrition, and health. The endocrine glands perform their task by secreting *hormones*, chemical messengers that travel through the body to stimulate some other part into action. They also control the growth and development of children's bodies, determine when men and women are able to have children, help build or repair muscle tissue—in short, they regulate what the body does and when.

Likewise, chemicals called *neurotransmitters* enable people to do things and, more important, to think about what they want to do. All nerve cells, whether in the brain or in the fingertips, exchange signals across a tiny gap called a *synapse* using more than 300 different neurotransmitters. When one nerve cell picks up a neurotransmitter that another cell releases, an electric charge runs through the cell, stimulating it to release a similar chemical. Different neurotransmitters exist for different types of stimuli: *endorphins*, for example, are associated with learning, memory, mood, and the ability to withstand pain, while *acetylcholine* seems to transfer impulses from nerve cells to muscles and the endorphin glands.

Humans' ability to produce these chemicals is not unlimited, nor even guaranteed. With age, various glands and cells slow down their production of hormones and neurotransmitters, and may stop functioning altogether. Illness or genetic defects also can interfere with the levels of these chemicals, causing maladies such as diabetes or depression. Finding natural or synthetically produced replacements for these chemicals was one of the great medical advances of the 20th century. In the process, the scientists who identified these replacements helped free countless millions of people from limitations imposed on them by their own bodies.

Running on Empty

For most of human history, the diagnosis of *diabetes mellitus* was a death sentence. Two thousand years ago, a Greek physician described diabetes as a "melting down of the flesh and limbs into urine. . . . The patient is short-lived for the melting is rapid, the death speedy. Moreover, life is disgusting and painful, thirst unquenchable, drinking excessive." In fact, the word "diabetes" is Greek for "siphon"; it referred to the frequent urination that the malady causes. The Romans added the word *mellitus*, meaning "sweet as honey," when they noticed that bees swarmed to the sugar-rich urine of diabetes patients.

Until the 20th century, physicians believed that diabetes was another disease for which they did not have a cure. These days, we know that diabetes really is a disorder, a malfunction of the pancreas, an organ that mainly produces digestive juices. Inside the pancreas are small patches of cells called the islets of Langerhans, which secrete a hormone called *insulin*. Insulin regulates the level of sugar in the blood and helps transfer sugar into cells, which use it for energy. When blood sugar levels rise, the islets secrete more insulin. When blood sugar drops, insulin secretion stops, and the liver releases sugar that it has stored into the blood.

It is a delicate balancing act. When there is too little insulin, sugar—specifically, glucose—piles up in the blood and passes out of the body in the urine. As a result, diabetics get little use from the food they have eaten. They get thinner and thirstier, as they need enormous amounts of water to flush out the excess sugar. These days, diabetics can inject themselves with synthetically produced insulin to counteract the failure of the pancreas, but there still is no cure for the condition.

The pancreas is an organ that does double duty, serving as part of both the digestive system and the endocrine system. The heart, the stomach, the small intestine, the kidneys, and some of the genitals (ovaries in women, testicles in men) also contribute hormones in addition to performing their major duties. Other organs, the endocrine glands, produce hormones as their prime function. These glands include the pineal, the pituitary, and the hypothalamus in the brain; the thyroids and parathyroids in the throat; and the adrenals, which sit on top of the kidneys.

Losing these hormones can be traumatic. Decreased levels of the sex hormones contribute to many maladies, such as muscle loss and *osteoporosis* (the thinning and weakening of bones) that also are seen in old age. Problems in the pituitary gland can cause abnormal growth, while an underproduction of thyroid hormones leads to a decline in physical and mental abilities, among other problems. It can be difficult, if not impossible, to adjust to a lack of hormones. For instance, until the 1930s the only treatment for diabetes was a nearly starvation-level diet that reduced the amount of sugars people ate to a bare minimum.

Likewise, it was very difficult for people to adjust to abnormally low or high levels of neurotransmitters, especially the ones responsible for regulating moods, emotions, and perceptions. Just as too little or too much of a hormone makes the body act abnormally, neurotransmitter imbalances cause many of the mental illnesses—from *depression* to *schizophrenia*—that plague a sizeable portion of the population. For centuries, people considered mental problems as something apart from the rest of medical care. Many cultures attributed insanity to visitations from gods, possession by demons, curses leveled at especially wicked or unclean people, or unfit family life. Some people affected by less-serious mental illnesses drifted, without really being aware they were doing so, into various forms of self-medication. Unfortunately, the most frequent form of self-medication was alcohol, which ultimately made the problem worse.

No one knew until well into the 20th century that mental illness often was a symptom caused by an imbalance in neurotransmitters. When nerve cells, or *neurons*, produce too little of a neurotransmitter, the brain cannot keep its activity up to normal levels: People's moods drop and their ability to think slows. When there is an excess of neurotransmitters, neurons send too many signals for the brain to process, creating an overactive state called *mania*. Depending on the type of neurons affected, people could hear voices in their heads, believe themselves to be gods, or shut themselves away in fear of having to interact with others.

Hormones and neurotransmitters alike were elusive chemicals to track down and difficult compounds to produce as drugs. It took a good deal of persistence and luck to create the medicines that people use to make up the difference between what they need and what they have.

Hormones as Drugs

Dr. Frederick Banting's discovery of insulin must have been one of the shortest successful research projects ever launched. Many scientists had tried to find the elusive hormone before Banting tried in the 1920s. They knew it existed because experiments had shown that it had to exist, and they knew it came from the pancreas because people or animals who lost these organs became diabetic. They also knew that if they could isolate insulin in animals and find a way to produce it in large quantities, they might be able to help diabetics regain control over their blood sugar levels. Until Banting's attempt, though, no one had succeeded: the digestive juices in the pancreas dissolved insulin too rapidly for the hormone to be extracted, and no one had been able to isolate the chemical in the blood.

It was possible to extract other hormones from humans and animals. A couple of decades before, three researchers had isolated a small number of hormones. Working separately, American pharmacologist John Jacob Abel in 1897 and Japanese endocrinologist Jokichi Takamine in 1900 produced pure samples of the stress hormone adrenaline, also known as epinephrine. In 1915 the American biochemist Edward Kendall extracted thyroxine, one of the thyroid hormones. Other researchers in the 1920s were focusing on the adrenal glands, the source of hormones that enable the body to deal with stress. But few, if any, researchers were trying to isolate insulin.

A private physician and a part-time physiology instructor at the University of Western Ontario Medical School, Banting was reviewing notes on the pancreas when he came across an article that suggested a solution to the problem of extracting insulin. The article said that tying off the *duct*, or tube, that carries digestive juices to the intestines would cause the

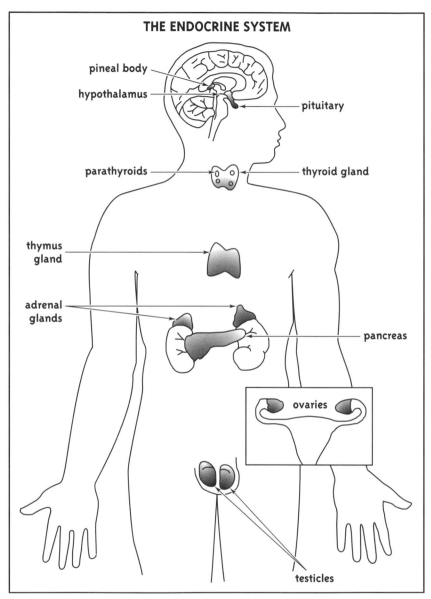

THE ENDOCRINE SYSTEM

pineal body

hypothalamus

pituitary

parathyroids

thyroid gland

thymus gland

adrenal glands

pancreas

ovaries

testicles

The human endocrine system normally produces the hormones people need to live. When a part of this system shuts down, whether from age or from a condition such as diabetes, people can make up the lack with synthetically produced replacements.

pancreas to shrivel. Banting was sure that if he carried out this procedure and ground up the dried pancreas, there would be no digestive juices to destroy the insulin, and he would be able to extract the hormone.

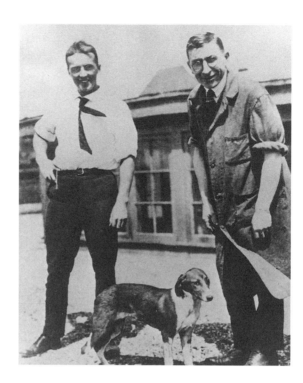

Dr. Frederick Banting and Charles Best with Marjorie, the subject of the 1921 experiment that proved the existence of insulin. (Courtesy Eli Lilly and Company)

Because his school had no money for this sort of research, Banting went to see Dr. John Macleod, the head of the physiology department at the University of Toronto and an expert on diabetes. Initially, Macleod was not interested in giving Banting the space, equipment, and money he needed to conduct the experiment. Banting persisted, though, and Macleod eventually agreed, giving Banting a small laboratory to use during the summer of 1921 and some money to buy a few experimental dogs. Macleod also put Banting in touch with Charles Best, a 21-year-old ex-soldier who was going to enter medical school in the fall, who agreed to work as Banting's research assistant.

Working together, Banting and Best performed the tie-off procedure on two dogs, which were always treated like favorite pets. During the day, they roamed free in the lab. When Banting operated, the dogs were under anesthetic, and they received the kind of care any human patient would receive while they recovered. Their first attempt to tie off a dog's pancreas failed: the catgut Banting used to close the duct disintegrated before the gland dried up. Switching to silk thread, the researchers tied off the duct of a dog named Marjorie, which developed diabetes within a few weeks. They removed the pancreas and dissolved it in a salt solution, coming up with a compound they called iletin.

When they gave Marjorie an injection of iletin, her symptoms cleared up within a few hours. Her blood sugar was normal, and there was no sugar in her urine.

Banting and Best had found a treatment for diabetes. But how long could they keep diabetic animals alive? More important, how long could they keep diabetic *humans* alive? How large an injection did someone need at a time, and how often did they need it? What would happen if someone overdosed? The two men kept running out of the drug, and they needed more in order to answer these questions. Then Banting had another idea. He had grown up on a farm, and he remembered that his father and other cattle ranchers bred their beef cattle shortly before they went to the slaughterhouse, because pregnant cows ate more and put on weight. Banting wanted the pancreas glands from the fetal (unborn) calves. It seems gruesome, but there was a practical reason for taking these pancreases: They do not secrete digestive juice until after the fourth month of development, but they do produce insulin. Going to area slaughterhouses, Banting and Best collected the fetal pancreases that would otherwise have been thrown away and used them in their work.

Eventually, the two researchers injected each other with iletin to see if the drug was safe for humans. By this time, Macleod returned from a summer vacation and was astounded at what the two had accomplished. However, he insisted on changing the name of the hormone extract to insulin, as the word was easier to say and other researchers had used it. He also added two biochemists, E. C. Noble and James Collip, to the team to work on purifying and standardizing the hormone. In November 1921, just six months after the project began, Banting and Best presented their discovery at a scientific meeting in Toronto. The next month, Banting read a paper about insulin to the American Physiological Society in Connecticut. News of insulin's magic spread quickly, but it also created problems for the researchers. Banting had added Macleod's name to the team's work in order to present the paper to the physiological society: Macleod was a member, and adding his name was the only way Banting was able to present the paper. That addition, as well as news reports on speeches Macleod gave about insulin, created the impression that Macleod made the discovery.

Despite this problem of publicity, and Banting's fury when he and Macleod won a Nobel Prize in medicine and physiology in 1923 that ignored Charles Best, insulin joined the ranks of miracle drugs that would include sulfa drugs and penicillin. Doctors everywhere wanted a supply of insulin to treat their patients. The Connaught Laboratories in Canada, near the University of Toronto, and the Eli Lilly Company in the United

States began making the drug, setting up entire production lines devoted solely to producing insulin. Banting and Best did not get rich from their discovery, though. Refusing to patent the drug in their names, they turned over the rights to insulin to the University of Toronto, which used the funds from licensing production rights to pay for more research.

Drug makers went through huge amounts of pancreases to make insulin in those early years. For each ounce, a laboratory processed the glands of 6,000 cattle or 24,000 hogs (which later research revealed also could provide human-compatible insulin). Today, though some insulin still comes from cattle or hog pancreases, much more comes from genetically engineered bacteria. DNA is deoxyribonucleic acid, the material that contains the genetic information in the chromosomes of all living things. It holds the chemical blueprint that determines what each cell of an organism will become, how it will work, and what it will look like. In a technique called recombining, scientists remove a piece of DNA from one organism and place it in the DNA of another. When the recombined DNA molecule reproduces, it passes along the genetic information in the DNA of both organisms.

In harnessing this technique of recombinant DNA to insulin production, drug makers splice a human insulin-making gene into a common, one-celled bacterium called *Escherichia coli.* They grow the

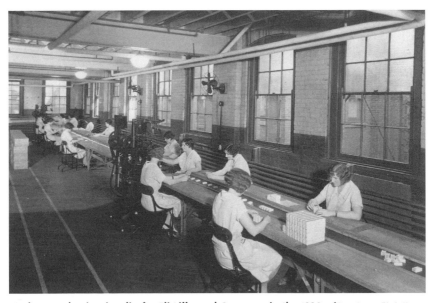

Workers packaging insulin for Eli Lilly and Company in the 1920s [Courtesy Eli Lilly and Company]

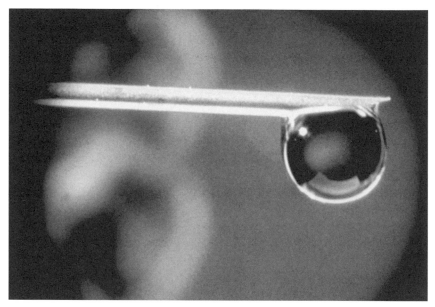

This is the first drop of insulin manufactured by Eli Lilly and Company. [Courtesy Eli Lilly and Company]

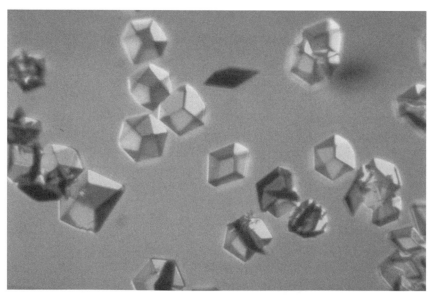

These days, manufactured insulin comes from recombinant DNA technology. [Courtesy Eli Lilly and Company]

engineered bacterium in huge vats, where they double their number every 20 minutes, multiplying by the millions and making insulin as the spliced gene directs. Producing insulin in this way is much faster and less expensive than getting it from animal pancreases. Better still, the insulin is always the same, never varying in quality and potency.

Banting and Best's success seemed to usher in a period of remarkable growth in the discovery of human hormones. Some researchers pursued the sex hormones, isolating estrone and progesterone, two of the female sex hormones, in 1929 and 1934, respectively. The discovery of testosterone, the main male hormone, came in 1935. At the same time, researchers became a little too eager to find hormone drugs that would be equal to insulin in treating once-untreatable maladies. A derivative of female hormones called diethylstilbestrol, or DES, appeared in 1938 as an easily produced antimiscarriage drug. Doctors around the world eagerly began prescribing the drug. However, taking DES turned out to have an unforeseen consequence: the drug caused an increase in some types of cancer and other problems in women's reproductive organs, as well as in their children's.

On the other hand, a hormone-based contraceptive—norethindrone, a progestin drug—successfully and more or less safely interrupted the monthly reproductive cycle. It and a later drug, a combination of progestin and estrogen that became known as *the Pill*, gave women a level of control over their reproductive system they had never had before. In turn, the Pill became a central feature of the women's liberation movement of the 1960s and 1970s and led to a radical shift in the social fabric of modern society.

In the 80 years after Banting and Best ground up dog and cattle pancreases for insulin, scientists have developed easier and more efficient means of producing needed hormones. For instance, the endocrine system in some children and young adults—roughly 10,000 in the United States alone—fails to produce enough hormones to produce normal growth. Not too many years ago, the only way to get human growth hormone was to take it from the pituitary glands in the brains of dead human bodies—the fresher, the better. It was so expensive and difficult to harvest this chemical that every bit of it went right to children whose bodies did not make enough of their own. Even so, there was barely enough. These days, though, the hormone is plentiful because the gene for making it was spliced into a number of cells, including *E. coli* and mouse cells, which reproduced and made the hormone. A Swiss company, Aries-Serono, that was seeking a safer method of making the hormone, developed the mouse-cell method. *E. coli* is a bacterium, and the insulin it produced carried the risk of triggering the body's immune system to reject it. Because mice, like humans, are mammals, the Swiss company's researchers reasoned that insulin from mouse cells would be less likely to cause that reaction.

Similar techniques have gone into producing estrogen and progesterone supplements for women who have gone through menopause, the point at which the reproductive system naturally ceases to work. This process is one of intense hormonal swings that cause *hot flashes*, irritability, and other reactions; it also leaves women vulnerable to health problems later in their lives. Once derived from animal sources, female hormones now come from synthetic production lines that—like those which produce insulin, growth hormones, and other types of these regulatory chemicals—ensure consistent quality and prevent such problems as allergic reaction.

Fine-tuning the Brain

Treating mental illness was all but impossible until the 20th century. Seriously mentally ill people generally were locked up in prisons, confined to special *insane asylums* (which were not much better), or kept at home with family members who did everything possible to hide them from the neighbors. People with less severe problems, such as *bipolar disorder* or *clinical depression*, were often able to function in the everyday world, with their friends and colleagues considering them simply to be eccentric or moody. In the 19th and early 20th centuries, many physicians treated mental illness with surgery or *shock treatment*. Almost no one had any idea that these problems stemmed from a chemical imbalance in the brain.

The first drugs used to treat mental problems were the barbiturates, a group of sedatives discovered in the first two decades of the 20th century. The first of these was barbital, developed by German chemists Emil Fischer and Joseph von Mering in 1903, followed by phenobarbital in 1912. Next came tranquilizers such as reserpine, discovered in 1952 by Swiss chemists working for the Ciba pharmaceutical company. The chemists were seeking a drug that could combat high blood pressure, and they had chosen to analyze the roots of the *Rauwolfia serpentina* plant, which had been used as a folk remedy in India. The drug turned out to have a remarkable ability to calm people down, and it and the barbiturates helped control some mental disorders.

The mid-1950s and early 1960s saw the first of the modern *psychopharmacological* drugs, ones that were designed specifically to treat particular chemical imbalances in the brain. Most of these early psy-

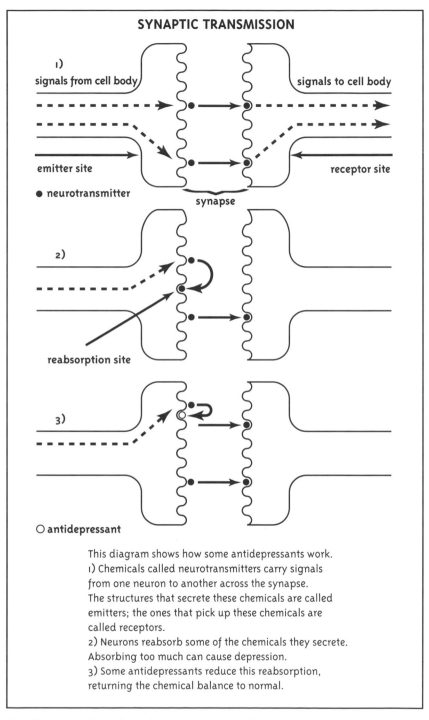

SYNAPTIC TRANSMISSION

1)
signals from cell body ......→ signals to cell body

emitter site   receptor site

• neurotransmitter
            synapse

2)

reabsorption site

3)

○ antidepressant

This diagram shows how some antidepressants work.
1) Chemicals called neurotransmitters carry signals
from one neuron to another across the synapse.
The structures that secrete these chemicals are called
emitters; the ones that pick up these chemicals are
called receptors.
2) Neurons reabsorb some of the chemicals they secrete.
Absorbing too much can cause depression.
3) Some antidepressants reduce this reabsorption,
returning the chemical balance to normal.

This illustration shows how chemicals carry signals from one brain cell to another
across the synapse. Many antidepressants and other psychoactive drugs speed up
or slow down the speed at which signals cross this gap.

chological drugs were designed either to calm down overactive brain cells or to counteract out-of-control anxiety. The first of these, chlorpromazine (also known by the brand name Thorazine), came out in 1954 as a drug to treat schizophrenia and other forms of *psychosis*. From 1955 to 1963, three antianxiety drugs—Miltown, Compazine, and Librium—achieved widespread use, which some people saw as an indication that modern life was too fast and too stressful. Other *antipsychotic* and *antianxiety* drugs have followed over the years, all of them the result of continued refinements of these sedating drugs.

More important for people who suffer depression, a series of drugs appeared that allowed physicians and psychiatrists to adjust the levels of neurotransmitters in their patients' brains. The first of these drugs, which came out in 1957, was the *antidepressant* imipramine, which increases the level of some neurotransmitters in the central nervous system. Normally, neurons reabsorb some of the chemicals they secrete to prevent overloading the brain with signals. In some people, neurons soak up too much of these chemicals, preventing signals from getting through. Imipramine and similar chemicals, known together as *tricyclic antidepressants*, slow down the reabsorption. A more recent type of antidepressants, *selective serotonin reuptake inhibitors* (SSRIs) increase the level of the mood-regulating neurotransmitter serotonin. Like tricyclic antidepressants, SSRIs interfere with this over-reabsorption, forcing the neurons to maintain a proper level of chemicals in the synapses. A third class, *monoamine oxidase inhibitors* or MAOIs, prevents the breakdown of neurotransmitters by a type of protein.

MIRACLES IN THE MEDICINE CABINET

People did not have to be seriously ill to benefit from the medical revolution of the 19th and 20th centuries. While antibiotics, vaccinations, and hormone treatments captured the headlines, other drugs quietly took their place in pharmacies and drugstores, not in the backroom laboratories where pharmacists worked, but out front where customers could take them off the shelves or ask a clerk to hand them over the sales counter. Unlike patent medicines, these drugs actually worked. And, as drugstores and governments gradually removed patent medicines from the marketplace, legitimate *over-the-counter*, or OTC, medicines became a respected part of everyday medicine. Today, OTC medicines are a multibillion-dollar industry.

Prescribing Your Own Pills

The main difference between drugs such as antibiotics and OTC medicines is the concept of *prescription*. A prescription is more than a written order telling a pharmacist to sell some drugs. It is a means of preventing people from taking drugs that either do not work on their disease or could kill them if they took too high a dosage. Most *prescription drugs* are too dangerous for people to use without the supervision of a physician, a dentist, or another highly trained health care professional, such as a *nurse practitioner.* Antibiotics, for instance, are not one-size-fits-all drugs. Some are effective against bacterial infections; others work against some types of fungus, protozoa, and even cancer cells.

Antibiotics also can be dangerous if used incorrectly. Stopping antibiotic treatment too soon, or taking antibiotics to treat diseases against which they have no effect, gives microbes the chance to evolve a natural resistance against these drugs. (Chapter 16 discusses drug resistance in detail.) Also, antibiotics often do not discriminate between hostile cells like disease bacteria and helpful cells, such as the *E. coli* bacteria that live in the intestines and aid digestion. Some types of antibiotics attack the body, causing problems ranging from deafness to kidney failure. Physicians use these antibiotics only if there is no alternative. Then there is the risk of an allergic reaction, especially to the 10 percent of the population that is allergic to penicillin and similar antibiotics. (Chapter 12 discusses these risks.)

Antibiotics are just one kind of drugs that pose such dangers. For examples, physicians and psychiatrists often prescribe lithium, in the form of lithium carbonate, to treat patients who have bipolar disorder. But an excess of lithium in the blood leads to brain or kidney damage, among other problems. Patients who are on the drug must check their lithium levels periodically to prevent this poisoning. Another class of dangerous drugs includes painkillers such as hydrocodone, most often sold under the brand name of Vicodin. These extremely powerful painkillers also are extremely addictive, and they must be prescribed only to patients who suffer serious pain.

OTCs, on the other hand, are powerful at low doses, avoiding most of the risks of overdose, inappropriate use, and addiction. OTCs usually treat the symptoms of a disease—runny noses, headaches, fevers—or other malady without attacking the cause. Some OTCs are former prescription drugs that proved themselves both effective and safe enough for general use. Sometimes, a drug's manufacturer will convert its product to an OTC form when it no longer has the exclusive right to produce that drug (as covered in Chapter 9). At other times, a manufacturer will produce a replacement for an existing prescription drug and will change the old drug's status to OTC to avoid competing with itself.

Other OTC drugs are produced specifically for the nonprescription-drug market. Analgesics, cold and flu remedies, antihistamines, indigestion drugs—essentially, any of the medicines sold on the public shelves of a drugstore—include pills and potions that give people the ability to treat minor problems without the expense of a visit to a physician's office. These drugs still have to meet safety standards, of course—the legacy of patent medicines and in particular of the drugs that killed people who thought they were buying treatments, but instead bought only tragedy. OTC manufacturers also must provide safeguards for their customers. Warning labels and instructions explain how people should use the drugs and when they should not be taken. Child-resistant packaging reduces the chance that very young children will make themselves sick, or worse, by taking medicine without supervision. And many cities and states require pharmacies to restrict sales of products such as nicotine gum or pseudoephedrine, which either can be abused themselves or can be used to make illegal addictive drugs.

But why do OTC medicines exist in the first place? Why not require prescriptions for all forms of medicine? The fact is that many medical problems are common enough that people can treat them without expert advice, and they simply do not require the heavy-duty treatment required for serious infections. A slight pollen allergy or a simple cold can cause a runny nose and make the eyes tear up, but the body can handle these ailments by itself over time. All that most people need is something to provide a little support to the immune system. For minor muscle injuries, simple painkillers can block the pain without problems until the body heals itself. By giving people the opportunity to find the appropriate treatment for their own minor ailments, OTC drugs help speed the process of healing.

Sneezes and Fevers

A majority of today's OTC drugs treat symptoms of allergies and head colds. Allergies are a malfunction of the immune system caused when the body forms antibodies to otherwise harmless substances called *allergens*, which can be such things as dust, pet hair, shellfish, or nuts. The reaction between the antibodies and the allergens triggers the release of chemicals such as *histamine*, which cause the symptoms that people with allergies suffer. The most serious allergies can trigger a reaction called *anaphylactic shock*, which includes a sudden drop in blood pressure, extreme breathing problems, and nausea. Unless treated rapidly with drugs such as the hormone epinephrine, an anaphylactic shock victim can die. With most allergies, though, people can handle their symptoms using an over-the-counter *antihistamine*.

Colds are viral infections of the mucous membranes in the nose, the throat, and the upper air passages in the lungs. Stuffy noses, fevers, sore throats, and muscle aches generally are the most serious symptoms, though some cases have progressed to serious, even fatal, pneumonia.

Antibiotics do not work on viruses and are useless against the more than 100 viruses that cause the roughly 100 million cases of the common cold that strike people in the United States alone every year. The huge number of cold viruses also explains why there is no reliable vaccine and why getting a cold once does not make a person immune. There simply are too many viruses to fit into one shot, too many for one person to develop an immunity against in one lifetime.

Fortunately, the hundreds of cold viruses, as well as the countless number of allergens in the world, cause a limited number of symptoms in the human body. Thus, cold and allergy drugs perform similar tasks. They dry up mucous membranes and relieve irritation in the nose and eyes by interfering with the chemical signals that create these reactions. They also shrink the membranes, making it easier to breathe. *Antihistamines* have been around since the early 1940s, when a French researcher named Bernard Halpern developed a method to synthesize chemicals that could neutralize the effect of histamines and promoted them as potential treatments for allergies. Researchers in the United States developed diphenhydramine, a commonly used antihistamine, in 1943. Others followed, and many of them became available over the counter, though most made the people who took them feel sleepy. Nondrowsy antihistamines came out starting in the late 1970s.

The one major difference between allergies and colds is that colds often trigger fevers in their victims. A fever is the body's attempt to kill a disease microbe by baking it to death and by speeding up the immune system. Unfortunately, extremely high fevers—those above 102 degrees Fahrenheit, or 38.9 degrees Centigrade—can kill brain cells or damage other organs. Counteracting this problem usually means turning to an antifever, or *antipyretic,* drug such as aspirin or acetaminophen.

Aspirin, in fact, is one of the most effective over-the-counter medicines. Ancient healers used a tea made from the bark of willow trees to reduce fevers and soothe aches, a technique that an English clergyman named Edward Stone wrote about in 1763. In a letter to the Royal Society, Stone wrote that he had experimented with the remedy for about five years and had identified *salicylic acid* as the chemical that contained the bark's healing power. Chemists in England and elsewhere in Europe tried to extract or produce a safe and effective form of the chemical without much success over the next 125 years. Finally, two German researchers who worked for the pharmaceutical firm Bayer perfected a technique for producing a nonirritating form of the chemical called *acetylsalicylic acid.* The drug went on sale under the brand name Bayer Aspirin as a prescription medication in 1905; later, it and a host of generic aspirin tablets entered the OTC market, and aspirin went on to become the best-selling drug in the world.

Pain and Swelling

Relaxation is the key to helping the body heal mild physical injuries such as pulled muscles and sprained ankles. Whenever there is any damage to a muscle or a joint, the body's natural tendency is to prevent any further damage by keeping that muscle or joint from moving. Even heavy exercise or physical labor counts as muscle damage, as prolonged activity stimulates the body to reinforce the muscles that have been used the most. Unfortunately, this tendency to inactivity causes a feedback loop between the brain and the muscles or joints, with the brain telling the body not to move to prevent further damage, and the body telling the brain that something is keeping it from moving normally.

Painkillers, also known as *analgesics*, interrupt this loop by dulling the signals from the injured muscles. *Narcotic analgesics* such as morphine, which are available only through prescriptions, essentially numb the central nervous system, preventing pain signals from reaching or registering properly in the brain. *Nonnarcotic analgesics* such as aspirin, ibuprofen, and acetaminophen prevent the body from producing a class of chemicals called *prostaglandins*, which seem to trigger nerve cells to generate signals of sensations such as pain or cold. So far, researchers do not know exactly why prostaglandins cause these problems or why analgesics are so effective at relieving the pain.

Swelling is another reaction to injury or infection. Just as the body will try to keep an injured joint from moving by locking the surrounding muscles, the immune system floods the site of an injury or an infection with blood, lymph, and other fluids. This response both isolates the site from the rest of the body and provides a heavy load of repair and disease-fighting cells. Unfortunately, the swelling also makes it harder for the affected part of the body to operate. Analgesics treat swelling the same way they treat fevers, by interrupting prostaglandin formation and shrinking blood vessels to their normal size. Without the pressure created by swelling, and with the improved circulation through the area, the body can heal the injury or infection more quickly.

Closely allied to antiallergy drugs and analgesics are motion sickness drugs such as dimenhydrinate (sold as Dramamine by the G. D. Searle Company, among other products). Dimenhydrinate is a combination of two antihistamines, diphenhydramine and chlorotheophylline, that also acts as a mild sedative. Researchers found that the antihistamine also blocked signals coming from the *vestibular apparatus*, a portion of the inner ear that creates a sense of balance. The vestibular apparatus is made up of three fluid-filled tubes called the semicircular canals, which make horizontal and vertical loops. As the head moves, the fluid shifts around, triggering nerve cells that send signals about this movement to the brain. In some people, the signals from the semicircular canals have trouble keeping up with changes in motion. Injury or illness can also trigger this reaction. In either case, the malfunction of these motion sensors can cause the symptoms of motion sickness. By blocking the signals, motion sickness drugs short-circuit these reactions.

Dieting and Diarrhea

Aside from aspirin and other painkillers, some of the best-selling OTC drugs are the ones that treat problems of the *gastrointestinal tract*, from the stomach to the end of the large intestine. *Indigestion, diarrhea*, and *constipation* are some of the most unpleasant ailments for people to deal with, and they have been part of human life for as long as people have been around. In many cases, these maladies are symptoms of more serious conditions—such as bacterial infections, parasites, or physiological problems—that require specialized treatment. Other episodes, though, are temporary, usually caused by such things as stress, a change in diet, or a short-lived illness.

For centuries, people treated these temporary episodes with various plant-derived remedies, most of which included some form of opium. In addition to numbing pain, opium calmed the muscles of the gastrointestinal tract and prevented it either from absorbing too much water (leading to constipation) or flushing water from the system (causing diarrhea). Even today, some OTC antidiarrhea medications use a nonaddictive chemical taken from opium to combat diarrhea. Nonnarcotic *laxatives* include *milk of magnesia*, a chemical also called magnesium hydroxide, and *mineral oil*, both of which lubricate the bowel walls and contents.

Counteracting indigestion usually is a task for *antacids*, pills and liquids that include compounds of calcium, aluminum, or magnesium. These compounds worked by neutralizing excessive digestive acids in the stomach. More recent OTC indigestion drugs, as well as some prescription drugs, function by interfering with the stomach's ability to secrete excessive acid in the first place.

One of the more popular OTC remedies for gastrointestinal problems, Procter & Gamble Company's Pepto-Bismol, started out as a treatment for infant diarrhea, which was responsible for many deaths in children younger than four years old. An unnamed doctor in New York State developed a mixture of pepsin (a digestive enzyme), bismuth salicylate (a metallic compound long known as an antidiarrhetic medicine), and other ingredients that halted the deadly symptoms of the disease. Because it did not contain opium, it became a popular treatment for a number of gastrointestinal problems in children, though its original manufacturer, Norwich Pharmaceutical Company, later promoted it as an upset-stomach cure for adults.

Even when the digestive system is working correctly, it can cause problems. People have been turning to prescription and nonprescription diet pills for decades to help fight the urge to overeat. As many as one out of every four people in the United States, and one out of every three Europeans, are considered *obese*, meaning they weigh 30 or more pounds more than their ideal maximum weight. People once considered extreme obesity simply to be a sign of moral weakness, although a "healthy portliness" was seen as a sign of prosperity. These days, medical researchers have shown that obesity can as easily be a problem of glandular malfunction or genetic predisposition as it could be the result of simply overeating. For serious weight problems—50 or more pounds above the ideal maximum weight—people sometimes pursue equally serious measures, such as *stomach stapling*, to cut down the amount of food they can eat. People who are trying to shed less weight often turn to diet pills.

Diet drugs have been a problematic part of medicine for more than half a century. Researchers at the R. J. Strassenburgh Company developed one of the first popular diet drugs, an *amphetamine* called phentermine hydrochloride. Like other types of amphetamines, phentermine forced the body into a metabolic overdrive, speeding up the rate at which the body used energy. The U.S. Food and Drug Administration (FDA) approved phentermine as a prescription drug in 1959, but because of its similarity to other amphetamines—also known as speed or uppers—the regulators put a limit of three months on how long a patient could take the drug.

Other prescription medications came out over the next few decades, the best-known of which was a combination of phentermine and another drug called fenfluramine, a product of the drug manufacturer A. H. Robins that combated hunger pangs by increasing the amount of serotonin in the brain. As a side effect, fenfluramine also slowed down the central nervous system, canceling negative effects of phentermine that included sleeplessness and anxiety; the phentermine in turn canceled out negative effects of fenfluramine such as drowsiness.

Unfortunately, as it turned out, this combination—called Fen-Phen—as well as dexfenfluramine, another diet drug that the FDA approved in the late 1980s, damaged the heart valves of many patients and caused an extreme rise in blood pressure in the artery that carries blood from the heart to the lungs. Following a number of studies that confirmed these often-fatal drawbacks, the FDA asked the companies that made these drugs to take them off the market. In the meantime, though, the drug phenylpropanolamine had become a popular alternative to prescription drugs in such OTC appetite suppressants as Dexatrim and Acutrim. The active ingredient in these products also was a key component in decongestants and prescription cough and cold drugs. As with the prescription medications, though, there was a serious negative effect. Studies of people who used phenylpropanolamine showed there was a small but noticeable connection between the drug and strokes: The FDA said that as many as 500 of the 10,000 cases of stroke each year could be connected to the drug.

There was no clear explanation for why the drug might be causing bleeding in the brain. In November 2000, though, the FDA advised the public to stop using prescription and nonprescription drugs that contained phenylpropanolamine and asked manufacturers to stop selling these products voluntarily. Because the drug already was classified as safe for public use and the connection between it and strokes was so small, the FDA could not force the manufacturers to take phenylpropanolamine off the market immediately. However, the agency began changing the drug's status in 2001 to remove its OTC status, restricting it to distribution only by a doctor's prescription.

Such reclassifications of OTC drugs, and of prescription drugs, happen frequently as researchers learn more about their effects. As the fate of Fen-Phen shows, drugs or combinations of drugs that may seem safe can turn out to have hidden dangers. Avoiding these unknown hazards is the main goal of the modern-day drug approval process, in which governments set up a path of experimentation that developers have to follow before they can put a drug, either prescription or OTC, on pharmacy shelves.

PART 3

On the Market

FROM THE LABORATORY TO THE PHARMACY

Where does a pharmaceutical company start when it sets out to make a new drug? How does a university biochemist decide to test a particular molecule to see if it can kill a microbe or heal a malfunctioning organ? And how does the public know that the drugs it gets are effective and safe?

In the United States, as in other nations, new drugs go through a strictly regulated process of research and testing, supervised by the FDA, before they go out on the market. The FDA has set the general pattern of drug development in America for decades. It constantly updates its requirements as time goes by and new techniques come into use. It also is a favorite target of drug industry lobbyists and health care consumer advocates alike, who criticize the agency for causing extreme regulatory delays in getting new drugs to market. It can take as long as 10 years for an experimental drug to gain approval for public use. However, this lengthy process came about as the result of a pharmaceutical horror that struck children across the planet.

Running the Regulatory Gauntlet

A drug called thalidomide changed the pharmaceutical business in the United States of America. Thalidomide was a nonprescription sleeping pill developed in West Germany in the early 1950s. Unlike other sleeping pills that contained addictive chemicals called barbiturates, thalidomide produced a deep, natural sleep with no risk of overdose. Some drug companies used low doses of thalidomide in aspirin and cough syrup as an added painkiller. Most dramatically, though, thalidomide canceled out a problem that virtually every pregnant woman experienced: morning sickness, the bouts of nausea that strike in the first months of pregnancy.

In January 1959 the William S. Merrell pharmaceutical company in the United States bought the rights to make thalidomide for the American and Canadian markets. By April 1961 Canadian doctors were able to prescribe thalidomide to their patients, and Merrell was expecting the U.S. FDA to approve the drug's distribution. However, the FDA investigator who was assigned to review the drug, Dr. Frances Kelsey, had doubts. Frightening reports were coming from Europe about babies being born with horrible defects—missing arms and legs, limbs shaped like flippers, and even worse deformities—to women who took

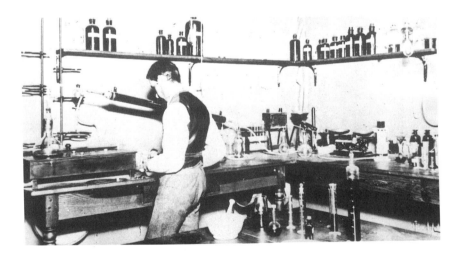

Ernest Eberhart was the first scientist in an Eli Lilly laboratory. In those days, it was not uncommon for a single scientist to conduct all the research work on a drug.
[Courtesy Eli Lilly and Company]

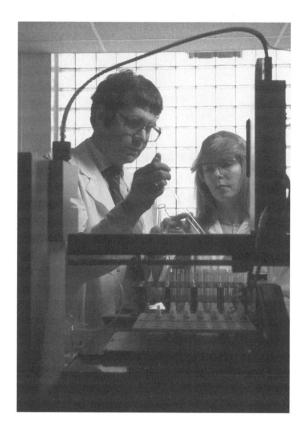

Today's pharmaceutical companies employ teams of scientists who discover and develop new products. [Courtesy Eli Lilly and Company]

the drug early in their pregnancy. Within days of each other in November 1961, West Germany and Great Britain took thalidomide off the market; other nations followed. The Merrell company told Canadian doctors to stop prescribing the drug to pregnant women or to any woman old enough to have a baby, but it still asked the FDA to continue reviewing its application.

Kelsey studied the data many times, finally deciding that the catastrophic birth defects were too great a risk. In Germany alone, thalidomide had been responsible for the births of more than 3,000 deformed babies between 1959 and 1962. Finally, in April 1962, Merrell withdrew its application. Thalidomide never went on sale in the United States, and the American population was spared the horror of seeing the drug's side effects firsthand. Later that year, President John F. Kennedy awarded Kelsey the Distinguished Federal Civilian Service Award for "her high ability and steadfast confidence in her professional decision."

But how could the German company that created thalidomide, and the American company that wanted to distribute it, develop a drug with such a serious detrimental effect? Simple. Thalidomide was a very effective sedative for all people and seemed to be safer than most other sleeping pills. Laboratory rats had been given high doses of thalidomide during safety tests, and none of them had developed any problems, including giving birth to deformed offspring. That was the problem. As it turned out, not even high doses of thalidomide produced birth defects in rats. Neither did thalidomide make the rats sleepy, as the records of the original tests of the drugs showed, which struck Kelsey as a sign that something had gone wrong in the testing. Why, she wondered, did the rats not get sleepy on such a supposedly great sleeping pill?

As it turned out, thalidomide had no effect at all on rats. Studies of the drug's effects on pregnant rabbits in the 1960s yielded deformities in baby rabbits similar to those in human babies, but by then these results were too late. If rabbits had been used rather than rats, perhaps the drug would have carried a warning and the tragedy would not have been as great.

Soon after Merrell withdrew its application, the U.S. government changed the procedures for approving new drugs. Pharmaceutical companies had to prove that their drugs were both effective and safe according to a stricter set of standards than in the past. Meeting these standards is a long, expensive process that starts in the laboratory, passes through years of animal and human testing, and requires researchers to file tons of paperwork. It can take as long as 10 years and up to $500 million to take a drug to market.

Unfortunately for researchers, there is no standard way to come up with a new drug. Each drug is the result of a unique process of discovery and experimentation; the only real feature they have in common is the scientific process their creators follow. When Paul Ehrlich, for example, was looking for a cure for syphilis, he knew that he needed to find an arsenic drug that would kill the syphilis spirochete. But he and his assistants tested 606 different arsenic compounds in hundreds of combinations before finding the one that worked.

Much the same thing takes place today. Even with advanced techniques for analyzing compounds and genetically engineering antibodies, modern pharmaceutical research largely consists of "mimicking natural products," of "screening likely chemicals, chance observations, astute questioning, and unexpected turns," to quote the American Chemical Society. When screening for possible drugs, chemists examine plants, fungi, animal cells, human cells, and other materials. This screening is a long, tedious process. Researchers do not always know what they will find, but they know they have a good chance of coming across something worthwhile.

One pharmaceutical company estimated that maybe 200 of every 2,000 compounds it studies—10 percent—will show some possibility of providing a useful drug. Of that group, maybe 20 will reach the testing stage—10 percent again—and only one might be found both effective and safe to use. In other words, less than one-tenth of 1 percent of a group of candidate compounds turns out to be something that physicians can use to treat patients. And that is an optimistic estimate. Other companies and industry experts have said that the number is closer to one in 10,000, which is $\frac{1}{100}$ of 1 percent.

After making a new drug, the pharmaceutical company has to find out if it works in humans before asking the FDA to review it. The first step, *preclinical testing*, determines if the drug is *biologically active*, if it is safe, and (most important) if it does what its creators want it to do. Over at least a year or two, researchers perform these tests on animals: first on rodents such as mice, rats, and hamsters; then on dogs; and finally on primates. Each type of animal is, genetically speaking, close to human beings, and a failure of the drug at any of these stages generally means it will fail in people.

After completing the animal studies, the drug's *sponsor* applies to the FDA for permission to start clinical trials in humans. A sponsor can be an individual, a corporation, even an agency of the government such as the National Cancer Institute or one of the other components of the National Institutes of Health. The sponsor files a form called an Investigational New Drug (IND) application, which provides such information as the chemical structure of the drug, its effects on the body, and the details of how it is manufactured. A drug is considered new if it meets one of the following conditions:

1. It contains a new substance, either an active ingredient or an inactive one (such as a coating).
2. It is a new combination of already-approved drugs.
3. It contains a new *formulation* or ratio of active ingredients already on the market.
4. It is an approved drug that a manufacturer wants approved for a new use.
5. It is an approved drug that a manufacturer wants to produce in a new form (in a liquid instead of in pills), in a different dosage, or for a longer or shorter duration of use.

DRUG DEVELOPMENT

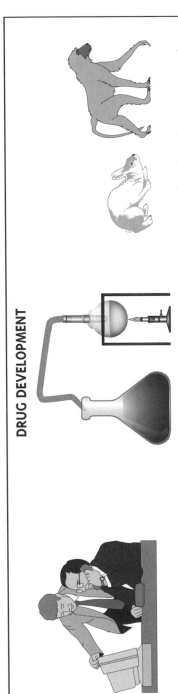

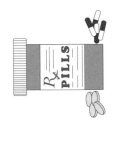

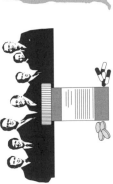

a) Drug company researchers identify a possible new medicine.

b) Researchers purify the drug and test it against microbes.

c) Preclinical testing on animals helps researchers evaluate the drug's safety.

d) If the drug is safe, the company asks the U.S. Food and Drug Administration for permission to test the drug on humans.

e) With FDA approval, drug company researchers put the drug through three phases of testing on human volunteers.

f) If human tests are successful, the company asks the FDA to approve the drug for sale.

g) If approved, the drug goes on the market.

The process of drug development, from laboratory to marketplace, follows this general pattern.

The FDA has 30 days in which to disprove the information on the IND, showing that the information provided is incorrect. If the drug maker does not hear from the agency, it moves on to test the drug in humans. Following these tests, which take place in three phases, the drug maker applies for final approval to make the drug commercially. If the drug passes its final review, it can go on the market.

Drug Testing

Starting in the 19th century, bacteriologists and other medical researchers grew bacteria in petri dishes and applied the chemicals they were testing directly to these organisms. But viruses can grow only in living cells, and it was not until the 1940s that someone found a way to grow live human cells that could serve as virus incubators. These days, initial drug screenings include testing chemicals on viruses and bacteria growing in human cell cultures. But testing chemicals in culture dishes and test tubes is not the same as testing them in a living organism, as the history of Prontosil showed. That drug killed bacteria in the human body only after its active ingredient, sulfanilamide, was released by enzymes within the body. In a test tube, Prontosil was ineffective. Actually, this reaction was unusual—ordinarily a potential drug performs excellently in the test tube stage, only to fail in animal or human trials.

Other complications do not appear in laboratory equipment. For instance, the chemical may not even get a chance to reach the disease organisms in a living body. If the drug is delivered by injection, other tissues may absorb the chemical and later release it to be excreted from the body. If taken by mouth, the chemical may pass through the digestive system without being absorbed into the bloodstream, or it may miss being broken down by the body's enzymes. Thus, researchers eventually have to test drugs in animals.

Using live animals to test drugs is emotionally and politically controversial. Animal rights organizations frequently protest against university and pharmaceutical company laboratories that use animals as part of their testing methods. To them, the discovery of new medicines does not justify caging animals and making them sick in order to test experimental drugs. Over the years, some extreme groups have burglarized medical research labs, stealing the test subjects (which these groups call liberation) and placing them with sympathetic families in other cities or states.

The opposing argument is that scientists worry about the stress and discomfort to their animals at least as much as, if not more than, animal-rights advocates do. This professional concern comes from the desire to make a drug test as accurate as possible, without interference from poor health, the physiological effects of stress, and the other effects of poor treatment. In addition, proponents argue, the fact that the work will end up saving human lives justifies the use of animals as test subjects.

However, scientists also realize the limitations of animal testing. As the thalidomide years showed, some drugs have no effect on some animals. Likewise, some animals simply do not get some diseases or develop other maladies. In the last two decades of the 20th century, researchers began developing methods for testing drugs that dramatically reduced the reliance on animal testing. The National Cancer Institute, for one, reduced the number of test animals it used by 95 percent when it switched to automated devices and computers that tested possible cancer-fighting drugs on human cancer cells, rather than on mice. Private-sector labs made similar advances.

Testing drugs in humans is less controversial because people volunteer to take part in these trials. The first set, or phase, of tests show if the drug is safe and how well people tolerate different doses. For this phase, drug companies pay up to 20 healthy men or women to take the drug and provide blood and other samples to find out how quickly the drug moves through the body. Since these Phase I tests measure only safety and absorption, test subjects do not have to have the disease. Phase II is where researchers find out if the drug is effective—if it performs as required, if it causes any side effects, and if the patients who receive it (between 20 and 100 in most cases) tolerate its effects.

The FDA requires two well-controlled studies for Phase III, using as many as 3,000 patients who have the disease or condition and who are in the care of fully qualified doctors in hospitals or clinics. These studies test the strength, safety, and effectiveness of drugs at different doses over a longer period. More importantly, they determine whether the drugs really are doing the job they need to do. In some cases, Phase III studies use *double-blind* or *placebo* tests, in which patients get either the test drug or a pill that contains nothing but sugar or starch. Neither the patients nor their physicians know who is getting the real drug and who is getting the placebo. In other tests, such as on antibiotics or cancer drugs, patients either receive the new drug or continue on the treatments they already use, again without knowing which one they have been given.

A drug for a common infection, which a patient would take for a couple of weeks at most, may race through all three phases in as little as two years. For drugs that patients might take for the rest of their lives, such as blood-pressure medications, the Phase III tests alone could last for the better part of a decade as scientists collect data on the drug's long-term effects. When researchers finally complete all this testing, they prepare and submit a New Drug Application (NDA) request to the FDA. The drug company sends all its information on the drug to the FDA's offices in Washington, D.C. It is not unusual for a company to ship the thousands of pages of data it collects for each drug via delivery truck. Then the company waits for the FDA's investigators to go through this information, occasionally asking questions about the drug's tests or its manufacturing process that the company has to answer.

Two or three years may pass before the FDA approves or turns down the application. Even if the drug makes it to market, the drug company must report to the FDA four times a year on how well the drug is working, where it has distributed the drug, and how it has been controlling quality. At the same time, a manufacturer can hold a *patent* on a new drug for only 17 years before competitors can make their own versions of it. In order to protect its manufacturing rights, a company usually applies for a patent during the first or second year of a new drug's development. However, it takes an average of 12 years to create and test each drug, meaning the company only has five years to make the drug without competition. Companies promote new drugs aggressively because they have only a few years in which to earn back the hundreds of millions of dollars they spend developing each of those drugs.

Generic and Orphan Drugs

When a pharmaceutical company's patent expires, other companies can make their own brands of those drugs or make *generic* versions. Generic drugs (also called store-brand or no-name drugs) have the same ingredients as brand-name drugs, meet the same safety standards as the brand-name drugs, and go through the same manufacturing process. The only difference between brand-name and generic drugs is in their effectiveness. FDA rules allow generics to be up to 20 percent more or less effective than the original drug. Since they are simply reconfigured versions of existing drugs, they do not have to go through the same testing process as new drugs.

Generic drugs are available for many prescription and nonprescription drugs, and generics can be much cheaper than the originals. Store-brand aspirin, for example, has the same ingredients and is made the same way as its brand-name competitors. However, it costs less because the consumer is not asked to pay for packaging, advertising, or added ingredients such as buffers or coatings. Throughout the United States and in most other nations, customers can ask pharmacists to fill their prescriptions with generic drugs rather than brand-name ones, unless their physician has ordered that the prescription be filled as written.

There are good reasons why a physician might not want his or her patients to take a generic drug, or one brand of drug rather than another. In some cases, a patient may need the exact strength of medicine in the brand-name drug, rather than the variable dosages in a generic version. In others, patients may be allergic or respond badly to the *inert* ingredients in a drug, such as the binders that hold a pill or tablet together, or the ingredients in a liquid medicine. Most of the time, though, generic medicines are more than adequate substitutes for brand-name drugs.

On the opposite side of the pharmaceutical spectrum from generics are *orphan drugs*. An orphan drug is one that treats a rare disease. About 2,000 diseases fall into this category, which the FDA defines as one that affects fewer than 200,000 Americans (less than one-tenth of 1 percent of the population). Like any other manufacturer, a drug company is in business to make money. But making a drug to treat a relative handful of people does not, in itself, financially justify the millions of dollars it costs to create that product. In January 1983 Congress passed the Orphan Drug Act, which gives pharmaceutical makers some help. They can claim a tax credit and apply for grants to pay for some of their research costs if they make an orphan drug. They also receive seven years' exclusive use of the drug, regardless of how long their patents have left to run, during which time no one else may sell it in the United States. These concessions encourage drug makers to produce medicines they otherwise could not afford to make.

A Case in Point: The Response to HIV/AIDS

There are a few exceptions to the standard drug-approval process. Sometimes the government allows a drug to jump ahead of the line and rush through the inspection process. Patients dying from *acquired immunodeficiency syndrome* (AIDS), cancer, or rare diseases are willing to try anything to get better, even experimental drugs that have not been thoroughly tested. Even so, these exceptions to the rules generally follow the same pattern of development of other drugs.

One example of this use of unapproved drugs came in the late 1980s, when the FDA speeded up the investigation of potential AIDS drugs such as azidothymidine, also known as AZT. AZT had not been intended as an AIDS drug. Designed to treat cancer, it was not very effective, and its creators set it aside until someone decided to see if it would be useful against the *human immunodeficiency virus* (HIV), which causes AIDS. Because people who developed active cases of AIDS were unlikely to live longer than a few years, many groups pressured the FDA to allow AZT's use before it had passed what could have been a decade-long testing period. On March 20, 1987, the agency approved AZT as the first safe and effective drug for helping some patients with AIDS and advanced AIDS-related disorders. It was the shortest review on record, taking place in less than four months.

To push through the study and to grant permission for patients to use unapproved drugs, the FDA created a new classification called *compassionate* or *treatment Investigational New Drugs* (INDs). AZT was just the first AIDS drug to receive this status. In October 1991 the FDA approved a drug called ddI (dideoxyinosine) for patients not helped by AZT. Even before clinical trials were finished, more than 22,000 Americans with AIDS received ddI at no cost. A similar thing happened with a new class of drugs called *protease inhibitors*, which blocked the function of an enzyme produced by HIV.

However, none of these drugs is a cure for AIDS, nor are they without their drawbacks. AZT in particular has serious side effects, including a severe form of anemia that often requires blood transfusions. Also, HIV can become resistant to these drugs very quickly unless patients take them in combinations that have been nicknamed *cocktails*. As Dr. Frank Young, a former FDA commissioner, once said, "We want the public to know and understand that miracles don't happen overnight, that studies take years, not months, and that patients are best served by rigorous testing and careful review."

10

PRODUCING MODERN PILLS AND POTIONS

Pharmaceutical companies are factories that produce chemical compounds rather than cars or computers. Like any other modern factory, drug factories have assembly lines that take in raw materials at one end and send out finished products at the other. A visitor to one of these plants will see workers operating machinery at computerized control panels, wheeling containers from one section of the factory to another, and watching over packaging lines to ward against malfunctions. Occasionally, a worker will remove a sample of the drugs being made and send it to a company laboratory for quality control analysis. And, of course, the company will stop running the line periodically to clean the equipment and repair or replace worn-out components.

Each industry has its own quirks or a specific way of doing things. The pharmaceutical industry is no different—though its quirks include using living things to create chemicals that improve the health of other living things. Details such as these, and the fact that its products are intended to alter living cells within the human body, have led to the pharmaceutical industry being one of the most closely regulated industries in the world. Government inspectors from agencies such as the FDA constantly inspect drug factories to ensure these companies are making drugs that are safe, that work correctly, and that prevent patients from being exposed to any potentially harmful contaminants.

Pharmaceutical Assembly Lines

Just as car and computer assembly lines developed from the need to make products more rapidly, pharmaceutical plants grew into their present form as drug makers tried to keep up with the ever-growing demand for their wares. At the beginning of the 19th century, most medicines came from pharmacists who made batches of pills, syrups, and other drugs by hand. The only exceptions were patent medicines; "sealed earth" tablets that came from just a handful of legitimate sources; and a very few legitimate medicines like cough syrups that some pharmacists produced in large batches for widespread distribution.

None of these medicines, not even the legitimate ones, could be guaranteed to work. Even if a drug was effective when it left the shop, time and the stresses of travel easily could weaken its chemical structure. There was no such thing as "sell by" dating, nor were there guidelines for proper storage. As for quality control, even the best-intentioned manufacturer or pharmacist could not say that each batch of medicine was as good as the one before it. There were so many variables—the quality of ingredients, the time of year, even the skill of the assistants who helped prepare the drugs—that the best a pharmacist could do was ensure that each batch was prepared according to the same method.

This state of affairs began changing in the middle of the 19th century, along with the decline in the use of heroic therapies. Pharmacists began filling carefully formulated prescriptions designed to cure specific disorders, and they began buying simple machines that made their work faster and more accurate. Some of the first of these drug-making devices were barrel-shaped tumblers that produced pills in consistent shapes and sizes. As mentioned in Chapter 4, medical researchers greatly advanced the technology of pharmaceutical manufacturing starting in the 1840s by inventing gelatin capsules and pills that broke apart easily in the stomach, releasing medicine for the body to absorb. Still, by the beginning of the 20th century, neighborhood pharmacists compounded many of their customers' drugs in the preparation rooms of their stores. And pharmaceutical companies' factories were not much more advanced.

When compared to modern-day drug factories, the facilities of an early 20th-century drug company seem amazingly primitive. From start to finish, most medicines were made by hand. Some production rooms resembled old-time moonshine distilleries, complete with wooden kegs and crudely shaped metal stills that processed raw materials for drugs.

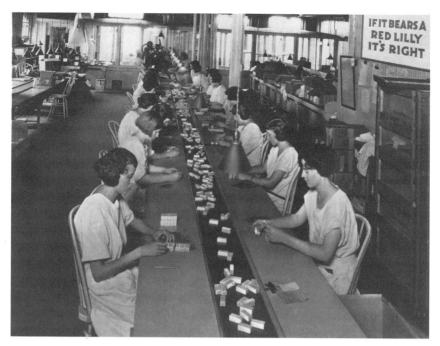

IF IT BEARS A
RED LILLY
IT'S RIGHT

This was one of the packaging lines at Eli Lilly from the first half of the twentieth century. Today, all pharmaceutical companies package their products on automated assembly lines. [Courtesy Eli Lilly and Company]

Other areas were no more sophisticated than a high-school chemistry classroom, with workers mixing chemicals at rows of lab benches. Young women and men filled pill bottles using specially designed, hand-operated dispensing funnels, while others packaged and labeled them, again by hand.

As medicinal knowledge improved, and governments continued to pass stricter regulations for drug makers, pharmaceutical firms improved their standards. In part, this move was a matter of image building. A gap remained between professional pharmacists and drug companies until well into the 20th century, probably because of the unsavory reputation of the patent-medicine industry. As recently as 1927, the American Society of Pharmacology and Experimental Therapeutics expelled members who went to work for pharmaceutical firms. This bias against drug companies started to change when manufacturers became involved in research and started discovering new drugs as well as making them. It also changed as drug companies automated their factories and took other steps to improve the quality of their products.

Modern drug factories have machinery that is much better than that available as recently as the 1950s. There are blenders for mixing ingredients, machines for forming pills, vats for cooking up some liquid medicines, and tubs for compounding others. What has changed most, though, is the amount of control companies have over the drug-making process. It is far easier to adjust and maintain temperature, mixing speeds, processing time, and other variables that make the difference between producing a safe, successful drug and making an ineffective clump of chemicals. At the same time, modern machinery is far more sanitary than the older equipment. Stainless steel tanks, connected by thousands of feet of pipeline, isolate drugs from the moment their ingredients go into the first mixer to the point where they emerge from their pill-forming machines or pour into their bottles.

Hatching Vaccines and Milking Bacteria

Some of the steps involved in making pharmaceuticals are a little odd. Since many modern drugs—such as vaccines, hormones, and antiviral drugs—are the natural products of living things, pharmaceutical companies incorporate many of these processes of life in their factories. Such techniques are not unique to the pharmaceutical industry. Bakeries harness the activity of yeast, a type of fungus that gives off a lot of carbon dioxide, when they use it to make bread dough rise. Beer and wine makers also use yeast, which turns sugars into alcohol during the fermentation process. In the petroleum industry, some researchers have been exploring ways to turn bacteria that eat oil into tools for cleaning up spills. And some museums use worms and beetles to clean the flesh from animal skeletons prior to studying them or putting them on display.

One of the most commonly used drugs produced with the aid of living cells is the influenza vaccine. Every year, health experts determine which three *strains*, or groupings, of flu viruses will post the greatest risk to public health. The flu virus changes very rapidly, and new strains develop from year to year. It is almost impossible to predict which strains will be the most active until people begin coming down with the flu. The analysis of past flu seasons and of early cases of the flu gives the experts a good shot at heading off the worst of these viral invaders.

In the United States, developing each year's new flu vaccine takes nearly a year. Starting in January, a group of immunologists and other

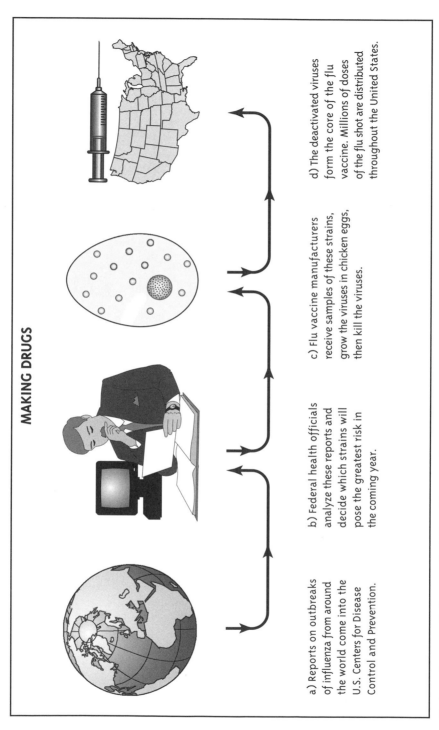

MAKING DRUGS

a) Reports on outbreaks of influenza from around the world come into the U.S. Centers for Disease Control and Prevention.

b) Federal health officials analyze these reports and decide which strains will pose the greatest risk in the coming year.

c) Flu vaccine manufacturers receive samples of these strains, grow the viruses in chicken eggs, then kill the viruses.

d) The deactivated viruses form the core of the flu vaccine. Millions of doses of the flu shot are distributed throughout the United States.

Modern pharmaceutical companies follow this general process when making vaccines and other drugs.

medical experts who work for the FDA determines which three flu strains will likely hit the nation in the following fall. These experts base their decision mostly on analyses of flu data from Asia and the South Pacific, where most flu strains seem to develop. Once the FDA has this information, it asks the federal Centers for Disease Control and Prevention, which maintains a collection of microbes collected from all around the world, to send over a batch of each virus for distribution to a small number of vaccine manufacturers.

Because vaccines are weakened or dead viruses, the manufacturers have to produce enough of the three strains for the entire United States. And because viruses will not grow in anything but living cells, the manufacturers need a long-living, and cheap, supply of cell tissue with the capacity to produce billions of viruses at a time. For decades, the common chicken has served as the source of this cell tissue. A fertilized chicken egg is, in essence, a single cell, with the yolk as its nucleus. Because viruses hijack cell nuclei and trick them into producing more viruses, injecting chicken eggs with flu viruses turns them into influenza generators. After a few weeks of incubation, the egg white teems with flu viruses. All the drug makers have to do is filter the viruses out of the egg whites, test them for such factors as potency, and combine the three strains into a single batch of vaccine. From then on, all that has to be done is packaging and distribution.

There are some risks in using methods like this to produce medicines. Flu vaccines contain a small amount of egg proteins, enough to trigger a reaction in people who are allergic to eggs and egg products. Likewise, the old method for producing insulin—separating it from the leftover pancreases of cattle and hogs slaughtered for food—can cause problems for diabetes patients. Their bodies simply cannot tolerate the chemical structure of those animals' hormones. And some patients have religious or philosophical objections to using products made from those animals. As mentioned in Chapter 7, drug makers have been using genetically engineered bacteria to produce synthetic insulin for diabetes patients since the late 1980s. Because the insulin that the bacteria produce is chemically identical to natural human insulin, there is virtually no risk of a negative physical reaction. Neither does this method conflict with religious dietary laws or with most personal desires to avoid animal products. In effect, genetic engineering has turned these bacteria into the medical equivalent of dairy herds, with the microbes as the cows and insulin as the milk they produce.

Real milk also has been the subject of pharmaceutical experimentation. Milk is a very potent, nutritious mix of protein, sugar, and immune system boosters (such as antibodies) that each species of mammal, over millions of years, has developed to feed its young and help prepare them to combat infections. Because mammals produce milk naturally and in large quantities, geneticists have spent decades searching for ways to "build" animals that can make medicinal milk. This way, the first step in manufacturing a needed drug would involve simply hooking up a cow, a goat, or some other farm animal to a milking machine. Research into this type of genetic engineering has gone slowly, but there have been some remarkable results.

For instance, in December 2001, researchers with the National Institute of Allergy and Infectious Diseases (NIAID) announced they had engineered a group of mice whose milk contained an antigen to the wormlike *Plasmodium* parasite that causes malaria. Malaria is a mix of high fever and severe chills, sometimes combined with anemia and jaundice, that develops when the parasite infects and breeds in the body's red blood cells. Throughout history, malaria has been one of the most lethal diseases that people face. It can be treated with drugs such as quinine, chloroquine, primaquine, and mefloquine, all of which came from research into an Inca cure for malaria that used the quinine-rich bark of the cinchona tree. However, people cannot develop a natural immunity to malaria, since the immune system cannot normally form antibodies against the parasite. As a result, the disease still affects more than 500 million people each year and kills more than 2,700,000.

The NIAID researchers reasoned that a properly constructed antigen that mimicked the chemical makeup of the parasite could stimulate the immune system into making the necessary antibodies. In their milk, the mice that the researchers engineered into existence reproduced the protein that makes up the skin of the parasite, giving the cells of the immune system something they could identify. The vaccine worked in laboratory monkeys, but it was not suitable for humans to use. To prove that their concept would work, the researchers had designed the medicine to be extremely powerful. This high-powered mouse milk was suitable for laboratory use, but it would take far more work to adapt it for medical use in people. But the researchers said that, with further research, it might be possible one day to breed goats or other livestock that created enough vaccine to protect entire continents against the disease.

Keeping Things Pure

Aside from making sure that drugs themselves are effective and pure, government regulators and pharmaceutical companies alike constantly monitor the factories that produce these drugs. In general, a pharmaceutical factory is a lot like a large bakery, a brewery, or any other large food-producing plant that makes goods for widespread distribution. Like food producers, drug companies make products that are ingested and have a chemical effect on the body. Unfortunately, factories are not inherently clean places. The amount of machinery, the level of the activity, and the sheer volume of space within any plant create a hygienic nightmare, requiring a constant effort to keep things sanitized. At the same time, factory workers have to battle mice, bugs, and other vermin (aside from the experimental ones in the company labs, of course) that could contaminate drugs at almost any stage of development.

At each stage of production, the machinery is kept isolated from its surroundings by at least a small stretch of bare concrete or tile flooring that can be cleaned easily. Workers usually wear plastic caps, gloves, and shoe coverings both to avoid contact with the chemicals they work with and to prevent dirt, hair, and other contaminants from mixing in with the drugs. Meeting the ideal of being "clean enough to eat off the floor" is the minimum goal in such a place, and in some plants even this level of cleanliness is too low. Drug companies make some of their most potent drugs under sterile conditions equal to those of microprocessor manufacturing plants. There are "clean rooms" in which workers must wear special masks and clothing that seal them off from the rest of the room, with their breathing air supplied through tubes and outgoing air being filtered before leaving the building.

Government officials periodically inspect drug companies to make sure they meet standards of cleanliness and keep their production lines in good working order. Under the Food, Drug, and Cosmetic Act, FDA inspectors can look over a manufacturer's factories, its warehouses, and any other buildings it operates, as well as its vehicles and "all pertinent equipment, finished and unfinished material, containers and labeling." The goal behind all this poking and prying is to prevent unscrupulous or simply sloppy companies from jeopardizing the public's health. Even with this monitoring, though, mistakes sometimes make their way through the system, requiring recalls of a particular batch of drugs or of all batches from a single factory. Rarer are acts of deliberate sabotage, such as a major scare in the early 1980s involving Tylenol, a brand of the painkiller and fever reducer acetaminophen. In September 1982, seven people died after an unknown person in Chicago, Illinois, contaminated a batch of Tylenol capsules with cyanide, a deadly poison. This incident, which led to a recall of more than 31 million capsules, heightened awareness of product tampering and contributed to the development of improved tamperproof product packaging.

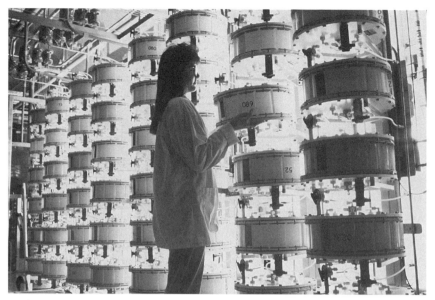

Modern pharmaceutical production, such as this insulin purification line, keeps as much distance as possible between drugs and people. [Courtesy Eli Lilly and Company]

Fortunately, incidents such as these are rare, and the world's pharmaceutical supplies are, for the most part, safe and reliable. In fact, medicines are so safe and reliable that people often forget just how powerful they are. Sometimes this lack of awareness can create problems, such as overdoses of OTC medications or misuse of prescription drugs. At other times, though, researchers and the public at large can be pleasantly surprised by a previously unknown ability of a commonly used medication.

11

NEW USES FOR OLD DRUGS

In the world of the medieval apothecary, the greatest medicines were those that treated the greatest number of ailments. Theriac, the all-purpose medicinal syrup, supposedly cured diseases, healed animal bites, and served as an antidote for poisons. People treated fevers, intestinal problems, and plague using terra sigillata. Whether or not these medications had any real effect was not important. Popular belief and centuries of tradition said such medications worked. Galen and Avicenna both had written about the healing powers of these materials. For a time, with no real methods of scientific investigation, no one could prove that the drugs were useless.

The idea of turning to one medical concoction or one healing technique to treat any malady maintained its attraction for centuries. George Washington's death following his treatment for a sore throat showed how risky this approach to medicine could be. And the concept of the magical, all-powerful elixir was one of the selling points that patent-medicine salesmen used to sell their mixtures of alcohol or opiates. Exploring the germ theory of disease and developing scientifically tested pharmaceuticals were part of the modern era's rejection of these primitive procedures and deceptive medications. Rather than providing universal cure-alls, physicians began matching specific drugs to specific diseases. At the same time, researchers began seeking ways to prove the effects of the drugs that pharmaceutical companies were making.

Naturally, no one objected when researchers found drugs like penicillin that were effective against a range of disease organisms. But the medical community was equally thrilled at the discovery of "magic bullet" drugs that treated only one disease, such as Salvarsan for syphilis or insulin for diabetes. In fact, if a drug seemed to be effective against too many ailments, it was viewed with suspicion until it proved itself with years of successful use, either in tests or as an approved medication. Part of the purpose of the modern drug approval process, in fact, is to limit the ways that drug companies can market new drugs. Pharmaceutical firms have to go through an entire testing program for each method of treatment they wish to have approved. Yet, drug laws in many countries, including the United States, allow physicians to prescribe drugs for other than approved uses, if the physician judges that the drugs will be safe and effective for the purpose. This flexibility in allowing alternate uses of established drugs has led to some astounding breakthroughs.

Aspirin: From Headaches to Heart Attacks

The transformation of aspirin from a simple headache remedy to a powerful heart-attack drug is an example of how even commonly used medicines can spark medical revolutions. In the early 1990s researchers found that taking aspirin may help prevent heart attacks in people who are at risk. In addition, they found that taking small doses of aspirin after having an attack can make recovery easier, and that taking aspirin *during* a heart attack can help people live through the experience. The truly amazing thing about these discoveries was that they involved the same aspirin tablets people could buy over the counter at drugstores, groceries, or convenience stores.

Until 1990 or so, people thought of aspirin as just an old, reliable antifever and painkiller drug that also, when added to water, helped keep cut flowers fresh a little longer. Aspirin prevented the cut stems from healing over, allowing more water to flow up the stem and keep the flower alive for a few days. In the 1970s researchers discovered that aspirin seemed to do a similar thing in the human body. In addition to reducing pain and fever, they found that aspirin prevents blood cells from *clotting*, or clumping together. After further research into this phenomenon during the 1970s and 1980s, a few groups of medical researchers started to wonder if this new knowledge could be used to treat heart attack patients.

Heart attacks are seizures of the heart muscle caused when too little blood reaches the heart. In addition to pumping blood through the rest of the body, the heart feeds its own cells through two blood vessels called the *coronary arteries*. Usually, heart attacks are the result of a buildup of fatty tissue on the walls of the coronary arteries, a condition called *coronary atherosclerosis*, a form of *arteriosclerosis*, or hardening of the arteries. Usually showing up in adults after their mid-40s, coronary atherosclerosis reduces the flow of blood through the arteries to a trickle, starving the heart muscle of oxygen. If the buildup becomes too thick, or if blood cells start to stick to the lining and begin clotting, it can shut off the flow entirely. From then on, a section of the heart starts to die, eventually causing the entire organ to shut down.

For years, only half the people who had a heart attack lived through it, and they were likely to die from a second or a third attack. Even when advanced surgical methods and simple techniques such as *cardiopulmonary resuscitation* (CPR) came into use, one of every three heart-attack victims still was likely to die before receiving medical care. The aspirin researchers thought that aspirin, with its ability to decrease pain and interfere with clotting, might be able to calm down the heart muscle and open up the blockage enough to get at least some blood through to the damaged area. It might even be possible, they thought, to save some of the dying tissue and increase the patient's chance of surviving.

To test this idea, the researchers set up studies at a number of hospitals and medical centers that received large numbers of heart attack patients. Each patient took an aspirin tablet, and the patients who survived their heart attack were told to take a tablet or a half-tablet regularly to prevent a second attack. Within a few years, the researchers had collected enough data to show that taking the over-the-counter headache drug right after a heart attack increases a patient's chance of surviving. Second and third waves of studies confirmed this previously unknown power of the common aspirin tablet. Better yet, other studies showed that taking a tablet or a half tablet every other day or so helped reduce the chance that men or women in some *risk groups* would suffer a heart attack in the first place.

Of course, the studies also showed there were some complications to this treatment. Aspirin's clot-dissolving power could cause health problems in someone who was taking blood-thinning medications or was at risk for other conditions such as a stroke—the rupture of a blood vessel in the brain. In addition, aspirin can irritate the lining of the stomach or cause other physiological problems over time. With a physician's supervision, though, taking aspirin as a preventative measure could be ultimately beneficial, the researchers said. In just a few years, doctors were prescribing aspirin as a means of warding off or recovering from heart attacks as a standard method of treatment.

More recently, researchers have been examining the effect of aspirin and other *nonsteroidal anti-inflammatory drugs*, such as ibuprofen, on colon, breast, and prostate cancer. These three forms of cancer began receiving a lot of attention in the 1980s and 1990s, mainly because more people were living long enough for these diseases to appear. Studies examining the lifestyles of people who were likely candidates for these forms of cancer revealed that men and women who took many over-the-counter painkillers seemed to be shielded from developing one of these tumors. No one at the beginning of the 21st century knew just why these drugs interfered with these forms of cancer; those answers would have to wait for further studies. But the ability to use these seemingly simple drugs as weapons against great diseases shows how drugs can have effects that go far beyond what their developers intended.

Going beyond the Design Specs

It is one thing to take an OTC drug to see if it works against a malady it was not intended to treat. It is a far more serious matter to perform similar experiments with prescription drugs, especially ones with potentially catastrophic side effects. Or is it?

Consider thalidomide, the sleeping pill and antinausea drug that caused horrific birth defects around the world in the late 1950s and early 1960s. There still were supplies of the drug here and there around the world after it was banned, including a large stockpile in the warehouses of the drug's manufacturer. Because thalidomide was an effective sedative, many hospitals used their dwindling supplies to help patients get the sleep they needed when other drugs failed to work. One of these hospitals was the Jerusalem Hospital for Hansen's disease in Israel, where a physician named Jacob Sheskin was treating an extremely ill patient.

Hansen's disease, also known as leprosy, is a bacterial infection that attacks the *peripheral nervous system*, the skin, and many of the internal organs. It can cause the skin to thicken and form lumps, and even fall off in large patches. Nerve damage can cause weakness in the hands and feet. Leprosy, which strikes up to 6 million people each year around the world, is not usually fatal. It often is painful, though, especially for the 60 percent of patients who are unlucky enough to develop a symptom called *erythema nodosum laprosum* (ENL), a pattern of extremely painful boils and sores all over the body. Unfortunately, there is no cure for leprosy, though physicians are able to control the disease with sulfa drugs and injections of morphine and other powerful painkillers. Sheskin's patient, though, was not responding to any of these treatments, and the doctor was desperate to find something that, at the very least, would help the man get some sleep for the first time in weeks.

Searching through the hospital's pharmacy, Sheskin found a left-over bottle of thalidomide pills and, not having any other options, started giving them to his patient. As Sheskin hoped, the pills overcame the pain of the ENL and his patient was able to sleep without inter-ruption. However, something else happened. After a couple of days on thalidomide, the patient's skin began healing and the pain of the lesions all but disappeared. As a test, Sheskin stopped the thalidomide treat-ments. Sure enough, the ENL symptoms reappeared, only to vanish again when the patient started taking the drug again. Sheskin gave thalidomide to a number of other patients with Hansen's disease who suffered the same complications, and they experienced equally dra-matic improvements.

Sheskin followed this discovery by repeating his work in Venezuela, where leprosy long has been a scourge on the population, and by con-tacting the company that made thalidomide to ask for some of the drug they had in their warehouses. Over the next decade, as news of this unexpected use for thalidomide spread around the world, various nations quietly allowed its return to hospitals and some pharmacy shelves, though only for use as a leprosy medicine. These nations gov-erned its use with a spate of extremely tight regulations to prevent pregnant women, or women in their childbearing years, from taking the drug. The U.S. Public Health Service, for instance, gave the drug only to patients in its leprosy treatment center in Louisiana. Unfortu-nately, these measures were not always successful, and a few women around the world gave birth to children with the same type of defor-mities as those born earlier. But the amazing success with using the drug to treat ENL—more than 92 percent of the patients who took thalidomide saw their symptoms vanish—spurred a drive to improve safety measures and keep the research going.

Throughout the 1970s and 1980s, a few nations allowed the com-passionate use of thalidomide, with most of the drugs coming from the German manufacturer's supplies. In the 1990s, though, researchers at a number of medical schools and hospitals in the United States found that the drug could treat *autoimmune diseases*, conditions in which the body comes under attack from its own immune system, as well as tuberculosis, some forms of cancer, and possibly even AIDS. But the FDA had not approved thalidomide for other than a limited number of uses since the early 1960s. How did the researchers get the chance to use thalidomide to treat these other conditions?

First, in the 1990s, a New Jersey drug company named Celgene Corporation had asked the FDA for permission to produce the drug in the United States and distribute it to leprosy patients who were not under the care of the staff at the Louisiana clinic. To make sure thalidomide did not cause any birth defects, Celgene and the FDA were to keep a close watch on all prescriptions for the drug. Physicians had to get a special license to prescribe the drug, and pharmacists had to keep detailed logs of who picked up each prescription. The government requires similar safeguards for narcotic drugs such as hydrocodone, to which patients easily can become addicted.

Of course, tuberculosis, autoimmune diseases, cancer, and AIDS are unrelated to leprosy. But this difference did not pose a problem once the FDA gave Celgene permission to produce the drug in 1998. Although the FDA approves drugs for only a limited number of uses, it also permits licensed physicians to prescribe an approved drug for any medical condition. These allowed but unapproved uses are called *off-label* uses, as they do not follow the list of treatment methods printed on the information label of every medicinal drug. Off-label uses give patients the benefit of new drug discoveries without having to wait years for official government approval. It also allows physicians to use their professional judgment to determine what treatments their patients need without interference, as long as physicians believe that their patients need a particular drug and that the drug will work effectively and safely against the patient's ailment.

When the FDA approved Celgene's request to produce thalidomide, it effectively made the drug available to any physician who wanted to prescribe it. Given the drug's history, not many doctors wanted to accept the risks that came with it. But some analyzed reports about thalidomide's effect against leprosy and thought the drug might have a similar ability to treat the diseases they were researching. Because of the ability to use the drug off label, these researchers were able to start tests on thalidomide that continued until well into the 21st century.

Searching for Beneficial Side Effects

There are drawbacks to using drugs for off-label purposes. One drawback is the risk that unscrupulous physicians will find ways around FDA safeguards and hand out addictive medicines, especially painkillers, to patients who become hooked on them. Even worse, a physician may prescribe drugs that are ineffective against a patient's illness, believing that the drugs have a hidden curative power that no one else has discovered. Such inappropriate prescriptions not only fail to help patients, but they can make some infectious diseases stronger, as Chapter 16 discusses. However, such abuses of the system are rare, and the benefits of allowing physicians to push beyond the boundaries of conventional treatment have proven to be worth the risk.

The trick is to identify drugs with the right side effects. Generally, the term *side effect* means a negative reaction to a drug, such as nausea, sleepiness, or dehydration. Part of the drug approval process involves finding out these side effects and comparing them to the reactions people have when taking placebos. All drugs have some sort of side effect, though these effects may not strike every patient who takes a particular drug. And some drugs may have hidden side effects that do not appear during standard studies but show up in real-world use. The discoveries of aspirin's ability to help people survive heart attacks and of thalidomide's ability to treat Hansen's disease were accidental. Aspirin came on the market long before modern drug-approval methods existed, so no one knew what it could do aside from cure aches and fevers. As for thalidomide, even if tests had discovered its effects on developing fetuses, no one would have thought of testing it specifically on leprosy patients.

There are better ways to push a drug's boundaries, though, than to rely on chance to reveal additional uses. Researchers will search through reports on existing drugs and other chemicals, searching for indications that one or another compound will cause a reaction that will attack a different disease than the one it was designed to fight. This work can have some surprising results. For example, in 2000 and 2001, a team of researchers at the Oklahoma Medical Research Foundation and the University of Oklahoma Health Sciences Center discovered that aspartame, an artificial sweetener, might help prevent or treat *sickle-cell anemia*. This genetic condition, which strikes people throughout the world but is most common in African Americans, causes the body to form red blood cells that are shaped like sickles or crescents. These mutated blood cells are less able to deliver oxygen, and they stick together easily, making them extremely likely to wedge against the walls of *capillaries*, causing painful blockages and leading to tissue and organ damage.

After reading that aspartame binds to a pair of proteins that help sickled cells stick together, the Oklahoma researchers added small amounts of the sweetener to test tubes of blood from sickle-cell patients. They found that one milligram of aspartame reduced the number of sickled cells in one millimeter of blood by nearly 50 percent, and that two milligrams of the sweetener healed even more of the malformed cells. The researchers then examined the blood of a small group of sickle-cell patients who ate or drank aspartame and found a similar decrease in the number of sickled cells.

As with many of these types of discoveries, the Oklahoma researchers stopped their work at this stage, published their information in a professional journal, and pointed out that their work showed there was room for further research. This procedure is common in scientific research, with scientists conducting preliminary proof-of-concept studies and presenting the results for other scientists to confirm or disprove. The Oklahoma researchers may continue their work in developing aspartame as a sickle-cell anemia medicine, or another group of scientists may take up the challenge and begin a series of full-scale pharmaceutical tests. If the chemical ends up as a treatment for the disorder, it will be just one of an ever-increasing number of drugs that started out as something utterly unrelated to its eventual medical fate.

12

WHEN DRUGS GO WRONG

Rabies vaccine, Salvarsan, insulin, sulfa drugs, antibiotics, polio vaccines—these and the other drugs that appeared in the 19th and 20th centuries completely reshaped people's expectations of medicine. For the first time, the public could get pharmaceuticals that could prevent or cure diseases without making patients feel worse than the illnesses they were trying to heal. Science, rather than philosophy or mysticism, became the foundation of modern medicine, and people started living longer as a result. They also grew to expect that even better chemical marvels would appear to cure any ailment.

As the world's experience with thalidomide showed, this faith in the power of pharmaceuticals has had its drawbacks. Though scientists and drug companies try to find all their creations' harmful side effects—if for no other reason than they are required to do so by government regulations—many drugs do not reveal their problems until after they clear the approval process. Sometimes, drugs create problems that appear only after years or decades of real-world use, longer than human volunteers take them during clinical trials. When these effects begin to appear, it can take years before they affect enough patients develop these problems to attract notice. At other times, one drug will turn out to interact badly with another in ways that researchers did not anticipate. Drugs even can interact badly with the body's immune system, resulting in mild to fatal allergies in those whom the drugs are supposed to save.

It would be nice to think that, with sufficient safeguards in place, only a handful of drugs would turn out to have these hidden traps in their chemical structure. Unfortunately, no system is perfect, especially systems that monitor chemical reactions in the human body. And while many researchers hope to tailor drugs to individual patients one day, it is unlikely that such error-proof drugs will be around anytime soon. Time, in fact, seems to be the only thing that guarantees a drug's downside will be revealed. A study published in the *Journal of the American Medical Association* in 2002 indicated that harmful side effects appear in many drugs only after they reach the marketplace. Reviewing drug warnings and recall notices issued by the FDA from 1975 to 1999, researchers discovered that more than 10 percent of the 548 drugs that made it through the approval process had to be taken off the shelves or given new warning labels. At least half of these drugs revealed their problems in seven years or less after going on the market. True, the discovery of the drugs' problems was due to the follow-up studies that the approval process requires, but in that time, millions of people in the United States alone were at risk of being harmed by these medications.

The Thalidomide Years

The story of thalidomide (as discussed in Chapter 9) remains the classic example of testing gone wrong and of how failing to detect a drug's side effects can have devastating results. Even though the painkiller/antinausea drug officially went off the market in 1962, its impact lasted for decades. More than 10,000 children were born with thalidomide defects, some of which were so severe that 2,000 did not survive their early years. The remaining 8,000 grew up having to deal with the various handicaps created by their exposure to the drug. In fact, when thalidomide was making its return as a drug to treat leprosy, a group of thalidomide survivors in Canada took part in the approval process to make sure no other children had to face the same problems they had.

Thalidomide's worldwide withdrawal in the early 1960s also reduced the level of awe toward and respect for pharmaceuticals that had grown since the 1930s. Medical science seemed to have taken control in the age-old battle between humankind and microbes, using drugs that were beating germs at their own game. The Salk and Sabin polio vaccinations that came out in the middle of the 1950s were the most dramatic example of how well things seemed to be going. Both versions of the vaccine served as a shield against a disease that crippled thousands of children every year. The only major problem with either scientist's drug had come from a batch of poorly prepared Salk vaccine, which infected 150 children with the disease. In contrast, millions of children in and outside the United States were spared the experience of polio.

The public admiration created by the success of the polio vaccine, and of other drugs that defended children against lethal diseases, contributed to the public revulsion against thalidomide. It was not just that the drug's side effects were so dramatic. It was that thalidomide had betrayed one of the basic principles of medicine: to do no harm. Drugs were supposed to make people feel better, not cause children to be born without normal arms and legs. Even worse was the fact that researchers could have discovered the dangers of thalidomide if they simply had conducted their laboratory tests with rabbits instead of rats. When the FDA and other nations' drug regulation agencies overhauled their requirements for drug approval, they shaped a process that would prevent future betrayals.

Some nations went a bit farther than others in protecting the public from dangerous drugs. The FDA in particular has been credited—though a number of health experts say it should be criticized—for having some of the toughest standards in the world. Drug testing can take a decade or more in America, years longer than in most European nations or in countries such as Japan and Australia. True, the FDA's process for approving new drugs, with its three phases of human testing in addition to multiple levels of laboratory tests, has filtered out many unsafe drugs. However, many patients, physicians, and politicians have complained about the time it takes to gain access to drugs that might cure previously untreatable diseases, even drugs that other nations already have approved. Defenders of the FDA system point out that the longer timeline provides a greater opportunity to catch any problems. Both sides, though, eventually have to admit that the only way to eliminate the threat of unsafe drugs is to stop approving new drugs altogether.

Why should this be? Why has it been impossible to develop drugs that do what they need to do without causing any other reaction, dangerous or otherwise? Part of the reason lies within the body. People are walking, talking chemical factories. Each organ, each cell consumes and produces hundreds of thousands of different chemicals from moment to moment. Adding any outside chemical to this mix, medicinal or otherwise, causes changes in how the cells and organs operate, and each person can react differently to the same dosage of the same drug. This variation makes it all but inevitable that every drug will create some side effects. While some of these changes will not be serious—drowsiness after taking some antihistamines or a dry mouth caused by antidepressants—the real danger begins when the drugs disrupt the body's normal operation.

Dangerous Interactions

The tetracyclines are a group of chemically similar antibiotics that were discovered starting in 1948. These drugs offered as close to an all-in-one treatment as people could hope. They could combat serious diseases such as the plague, typhus, and cholera, but they also could treat less-dangerous conditions such as acne and some upper respiratory tract infections. Better still, they seemed to have fewer side effects than penicillin or many other antibiotics. Large doses of tetracycline could cause serious liver and kidney damage, but at lower concentrations the antibiotics were generally safe. Medical researchers and government regulators, in fact, judged they were safe enough for growing children to take, offering parents and physicians a seemingly perfect weapon against the germs that circulated during the school year.

After a few years, though, dentists began noticing something odd. A lot of young people, especially those in their junior-high-school years, were showing up with strange-looking spots on their teeth. Normally, the tooth's *enamel*, or surface material, ranges in color from a milky white to a mellow ivory. These children, though, began developing beige spots in the center of their teeth. Investigating their patients' medical histories, the dentists soon discovered the source of the discoloration. All these children had taken tetracycline, often more than once, to treat a childhood illness. Somehow, the antibiotic had triggered a chemical change in the surface of the teeth that caused the discolorations.

The phenomenon a side effect that had not shown up while the drugs were being developed and tested. Researchers had discovered that large doses of a tetracycline could seriously damage the liver and kidneys, though physicians could avoid these and other dangers by carefully monitoring their patients and altering their antibiotics over time. These antibiotics were supposed to attack microbes inside the body, not the body itself, and no other antibiotic had shown such a reaction. Nevertheless, physicians stopped prescribing tetracyclines for children or pregnant women to prevent any other cases from cropping up.

Other drug reactions can be much worse. Take aspirin, for example—or, rather, do not take it during an attack of influenza, chicken pox, or other viral diseases. Aspirin has been around so long that people consider it as harmless as any drug could be. It is one of the first drugs people turn to when they develop fevers, headaches, or muscle aches. But in the 1960s medical researchers discovered that aspirin has a dark side. When children take aspirin to combat the effects of some viral infections, they are at greater risk of developing a disease called Reye's syndrome. This liver and nervous system disease, which can lead

NEGATIVE DRUG REACTIONS

Drug Type	Common Reactions	Treatment to Counter Reaction
penicillin – antibiotic – includes drugs such as amoxil and ampicillin	– mild rash that appears a few days after patient starts taking the drug – about 10 percent of people may go into anaphylactic shock	– antihistamine to fight rash; switch to a non-penicillin-based antibiotic – immediate injection of steroids if patient goes into shock
sulfa drugs – antibiotics – still prescribed to treat some illnesses	– mild to moderate rash, as with penicillin-based antibiotics	– antihistamine to fight rash; switch to a non-sulfa antibiotic
insulin – hormone drug used to treat diabetes – reactions appear in response to insulin from cattle and pigs	– itchy rash around site of injection; also may include hives, problems with breathing, and/or a faster heartbeat	– switch to purified insulin or insulin made with genetically engineered bacteria
iodine – used as a "contrast medium" to make blood vessels show up on X rays	– dizziness, hives, nausea, vomiting. – one in 1,000 people may go into anaphylactic shock	– if needed, medical staff can provide proper treatment, including steroids or other drugs to treat anaphylaxis

Some people simply cannot tolerate pharmaceutical drugs. This chart shows some of the more common allergic reactions and the means of counteracting them.

to brain damage or death, strikes children mostly from four to 15 years old after mild bouts of a viral illness. No one knows exactly why children develop this disease in the first place, or why aspirin makes it more likely they will come down with it. Knowing that aspirin can interact with an illness with such dramatic consequences, though, makes it less likely that children will develop this condition.

There are explanations for some of aspirin's other problematic side effects. For instance, aspirin bottles carry notices warning people not to take the drug if they already are taking anticoagulants or blood-thinning drugs to treat conditions such as heart disease. Aspirin is an anticoagulant (anticlotting drug) in its own right, and combining it with more powerful drugs can lead to uncontrollable bleeding. Physicians have to be very careful to avoid drug interactions such as these. For example, if a patient is taking an antidepressant or a prescription sleeping pill, his or her physician has to be careful about prescribing any medications that cause the body to retain water. Without the ability to flush excess medication from the body, patients can begin to overdose on their other drugs, hallucinating or developing other problems in how they perceive the world. Mistakes happen, though, which is why pharmacists check each patient's medications for conflicts.

Drug Allergies

Drugs need not interact with diseases or with other drugs to cause problems for patients. Many drugs can be dangerous all by themselves.

At the end of World War II, when antibiotics were revolutionizing medical care, doctors provided injections and wrote prescriptions for these wonder drugs as soon as they became available. Naturally, considering the fame it received for the millions of lives it saved during the war, penicillin was one of the most frequently prescribed antibiotics. But an alarming trend appeared as more people took the drug. For every nine people whose infections cleared up under the onslaught of penicillin, one person died soon after receiving the drug. The healing properties of penicillin did not mask the fact that the drug was, after all, a chemical and that some people's bodies simply could not handle it.

Few, if any, drugs will not trigger an allergic reaction in some people. With luck, the worst symptoms a patient will have to endure are things like rashes or mild fevers. The truly unfortunate will go into anaphylactic shock, the full-body reaction that can lead to brain damage or death if not counteracted quickly. These reactions may appear during a new drug's human trials in the volunteer base; if so, and if the number of people who are likely to be allergic seems small enough, the drug still can be approved. If the tests show that too many people will become allergic to the drug, it will not get approval, or it will be approved only for a very small group of patients.

Sometimes, a drug's allergic properties will be the result of the way it is made, rather than of the drug itself. As mentioned in Chapter 10, people who are allergic to eggs also will be allergic to influenza vaccines, which develop inside the whites of fertilized chicken eggs and which contain small amounts of egg proteins. Drugs derived from animal cells—such as hormones and some arthritis medicines—can cause reactions in people whose immune systems are set up to attack the proteins from those animals. The body also can develop sensitivity to mold-based drugs, such as antibiotics, and the few mineral-based drugs, like the antiseptic tincture iodine. Fortunately, there are alternatives to these allergy-causing drugs. Not only can patients substitute one type of drug for another, such as using acetaminophen instead of aspirin, but many drug makers synthesize versions of drugs that avoid these risks.

Expired Medications

Unlike the pull dates on food such as eggs or meat, drug expiration dates do not indicate when a prescription or an over-the-counter drug becomes dangerous to consume. Instead, they show how long drugs can be expected to retain their full strength. All drugs lose their potency over time, as their chemical structure slowly breaks down under the effects of temperature, *oxidation*, humidity, and similar environmental conditions. In the past, few people had any idea when it was time to get rid of a box of throat lozenges or a bottle of prescription cough medicine. Then, in 1978, the FDA ordered drug makers to include this information on the labels of every prescription drug and all but a few OTC medicines. The danger was not that an expired drug would sicken or kill someone who took it, but that people would not get the amount of medicine that they needed for their illness.

For an OTC drug like a cough drop or a decongestant, expiration dates simply were a means of ensuring that people were getting the full value of the drug they were buying. For prescription drugs, though, the situation was more serious. If patients received antibiotics that were at less than their full strength, they might find themselves still sick after taking the full course of the drug. Worse still, by attacking their bacteria with underpowered drugs, patients would help the germs become stronger and build resistance to the antibiotic. What started as a low-level contagion could develop into a far more serious, or even a deadly, infection that would require a more powerful antibiotic. Similar problems can pop up with other drugs. An underpowered dose of insulin could lead to a buildup of glucose in a diabetes patient's blood, precisely the condition that the hormone is designed to prevent.

Drug makers calculate expiration dates in much the same way that nuclear physicists determined the *half-life* of radioactive particles. An element's half-life is the time it takes for half of that element to break down, or *decay*, into a stable, nonradioactive form. Physicists determine an element's half-life by taking a sample and measuring how much of the material decays over a given period. They then calculate how long it would take for half of that sample to break down. Based on the drug's performance over a period of months or years, the researchers calculate how long it would take before the drug became too weak to have a useful effect. They then add in a safety margin and establish that figure as the drug's expiration date.

These calculations assume that most people will store their drugs properly, in areas that do not expose them to high temperatures, light, or high humidity. Each of these three factors drastically reduces most drugs' potency by breaking down their chemical bonds. The problem is that most people store their pharmaceutical and OTC drugs in a bathroom medicine chest or next to a sink, exposing them to both high temperature and high humidity (think of what a bathroom feels like following a long, hot shower). For drugs that people plan to take for only a few days to a couple of weeks, such conditions may not reduce the drug's effective life much, if at all. For longer-term prescriptions or OTC drugs that people plan to keep for a year or more, being exposed to these extremes can sap the medicines of their healing power.

PART 4

Alternative Treatments

BACK TO THE GARDEN?

The drive to find new and better medicines has taken scientists into the structure of living cells, into laboratories with petri dishes colonized by exotic molds, and into cyberspace, where computers analyze digitized chemical compounds to hit upon the world's next pharmaceutical magic bullet. In one form or another, this pattern of research has been in place since the early days of scientific pharmacology. In the last few decades of the 20th century, though, a growing number of medical researchers and physicians started reexamining an older style of medicine that had been pushed aside in much of the Western world.

Vaccines, antibiotics, and the rest of the modern chemical arsenal against disease did not just eliminate dangerous and fraudulent medicines. They also supplanted the old plant-based remedies that people had used for centuries, if not for millennia. These folk cures did not vanish, though. While countries such as the United States, Japan, and the nations of Europe led the revolution in lab-and-factory pharmaceutical development, many people continued to practice the traditional forms of medicine on which their ancestors relied, even in nations spearheading the drive to find new drugs through scientific means. These people had a good reason to hold onto the old knowledge. Many modern medicines came directly from ancient remedies: the antimalarial drug quinine was isolated from cinchona bark, for example, while the heart medicine digitalis had its source in the foxglove plant.

Researchers decided to experiment with other folk cures to see if they also contained potent, and marketable, healing chemicals. Many of the plants that the researchers studied were the same "simples" that ancient physicians had used and that medieval wise women had grown in their home gardens. Others were everyday herbs that people long ago recognized as having the ability to cure afflictions ranging from cuts to fevers. The laboratory-based search for unrecognized healing compounds also continued, with scientists analyzing natural materials that never had been used for healing purposes. But even this research proceeded in different directions than had been taken before.

Searching the Jungles
for Cancer Cures

For decades, scientists have been certain that Earth's jungles and tropical rain forests, with their vast numbers of plant and animal species, are home to hundreds of possible medicines. Pharmaceutical firms around the world have spent millions of dollars on expeditions to gather samples of these materials and take them back to their corporate laboratories for analysis. In the early 1990s, the drug manufacturer Merck, Sharp & Dohme (now known simply as Merck & Company, Inc.) signed a contract with Costa Rica to develop drugs from plants and animals found in the Central American nation's jungles. In exchange for a $1 million down payment and the promise of future payments, the company received the exclusive rights to collect samples of plant life, animal life, fungi, microbes, and anything else that might yield the active ingredients of new drugs.

Few other drug companies have gone to such extreme lengths to seek out the next great superdrugs. Yet, the lure of the jungle as a pharmaceutical treasure trove has drawn many biologists into extended journeys away from the comforts and conveniences of civilization. Perhaps the most idealized objective of these botanical expeditions is a cure for most, if not all, forms of cancer. Such a cure, scientists imagine, might hide within the seeds of a bush deep within the island of Borneo or in a flower growing high up in the *canopy* of the Amazon Basin rain forest. Given enough time and enough financial backing, researchers believe, they could harvest these *biochemical* riches.

In fact, it was a cancer cure that drew a great deal of attention to the fact that many powerful drugs were yet to be discovered. In a vast program to screen natural compounds for possible cancer-fighting drugs, scientists sponsored by the U.S. National Cancer Institute analyzed plants from the forests of the Pacific Northwest. One of the plants they tested was the Pacific yew tree, an evergreen whose bark contained a powerful chemical compound that the scientists dubbed *paclitaxel*, which the Bristol-Myers Squibb Company later marketed under the trade name Taxol. Paclitaxel not only shrank tumors, especially those of breast and ovarian cancer, but it killed cancer cells in a way that researchers never had seen before. All body cells, even cancer cells, reproduce by dividing into two identical *daughter cells*. Whenever a cell divides, it forms a sort of chemical scaffold that supports both halves as they pull apart and form cellular walls. Paclitaxel stops cells from forming these scaffolds, causing the cells to collapse.

Scientists first discovered paclitaxel in the early 1970s, but developing it into a usable drug took more than a decade. Taxol was not ready for clinical testing until the mid-1980s. Part of the delay came from the trouble it took to make enough of the drug to study. Supplying enough Taxol to treat one patient meant processing the bark from three yew trees that are at least four inches in diameter. It takes a yew tree from 70 to 100 years to reach that size, though, which already put a limit on how many patients could receive the drug. In 1991 the National Cancer Institute asked for enough paclitaxel to run tests on 12,500 patients, which meant cutting down 38,000 Pacific yews to get the 750,000 pounds of bark needed to extract the drug. At the time, lumber companies working in the Pacific Northwest could harvest this number of yew trees as part of their normal logging work. Yew trees were useless as timber, and lumber companies often burned off whole tracts of them to get to more valuable trees. On the other hand, cutting down the slow-growing yews for drugs could have caused their extinction very quickly, depriving the world of both the drug and the trees.

Fortunately, further research in the early 1990s revealed a way to gain the drug without losing the trees. At the University of Florida, a research chemist named Dr. Robert Holton decided to test other types of yew trees to see if they also contained paclitaxel. None did. However, he found that the needles of a shrub-sized yew—the English yew, which often is used for ornamental landscaping—contain a substance called baccatin III. By itself, baccatin III does not treat cancer, but it can be processed into paclitaxel. Using this sturdy shrub eliminated the need to cut down a full-sized yew tree for its bark. Better still, it takes only two pounds of needles to get the baccatin needed to make enough paclitaxel to treat a patient. Because the needles grow back as long as the shrub is alive, each English yew can yield multiple harvests.

Another possibility, of course, was to synthesize paclitaxel in a laboratory, which chemists tried to do for nearly a decade. The chemical's structure turned out to be so complex, though, that the chemists could not duplicate it using the technology that was available at the time. The only other option was to grow Pacific yew bark cells in the laboratory, using a similar type of tissue culturing used to grow skin cells. In culturing bark cells, laboratory technicians placed small pieces of bark in trays of nutrient-rich gel, in which the cells grew into a mass called a *callus*. Cells from the original calluses went to produce more cultures and more calluses over the next several weeks, after which the technicians dried some of the calluses and extracted the paclitaxel. Scientists still can extract small amounts of the drug this way. The method did not result in creating a forest's worth of paclitaxel-producing calluses, though. Most paclitaxel comes from processing English yew needles.

Herbs, Vitamins, and Mineral Pills

Perhaps the most astounding thing about paclitaxel's discovery was its extremely ordinary origin. Yew trees are neither exotic nor endangered, yet they produce chemicals that effectively combat two of the most serious diseases women face. Likewise, many seemingly unremarkable plants have been identified as possessing unusual healing properties. Herbalists—people who know the uses of plants for medicines and cosmetics—kept this knowledge alive even when laboratory-produced drugs took a dominant role in health care. In some nations, particularly those of Asia, physicians incorporated both traditional medicines and Western drugs as they treated patients. In other lands, herbalists became part of an alternative medical culture.

In the 1970s and 1980s, people began taking an interest in the work of herbalists and in the general subject of alternative medicine, and medical scientists started examining these centuries-old healing plants. It is difficult to say exactly why herbal remedies became so popular during this time. One reason might have been that people were becoming disenchanted both with the rising cost of modern medicine and with the side effects that accompany modern pharmaceuticals. At the same time, though, such social movements as the trend toward *organic farming* and the criticism and distrust of synthesized chemicals may also have made people more receptive to these alternative treatments. Whatever the cause, store shelves began filling up with such products as Saint-John's-wort, which was touted as a natural antidepressant, and echinacea, a flower that yielded a chemical that supposedly could prevent colds, or at least cut them short.

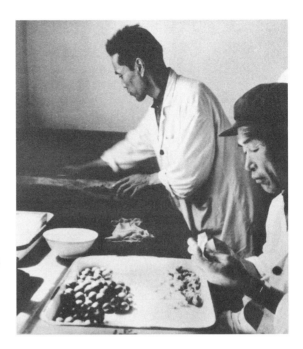

Traditional herbal medicines have been in use around the world for millennia. Here, herbalists prepare drugs in a 1950s Chinese hospital. [World Health Organization photo, courtesy of the National Library of Medicine]

In addition to herbal remedies, vitamin and mineral supplements became popular as people started exploring ways to prevent illness. Vitamins are catalysts for other chemical reactions in the human body, maintaining functions that range from the assembly of DNA molecules in cells to the creation of new skin over wounds and sores. Human beings need 13 vitamins in order to stay alive: Vitamin A, or retinol; eight vitamins known as the *B complex;* vitamin C, also called ascorbic acid; vitamin D, or cholecalciferol; vitamin E, or tocopherol; and vitamin K. Most people get almost all the vitamins that they need if they eat a healthy, balanced diet. The exceptions include three of the B vitamins: biotin, niacin, and pantothenic acid; vitamin K, which the intestinal bacteria produce; and vitamin D, which the skin makes when exposed to sunlight.

As catalysts, vitamins do not so much do things in the body as ensure that things get done. Vitamin A helps the body maintain the health of the eyes, the skin, the urinary tract, and the linings of various organ systems. Vitamin C allows the body to grow and replace various tissues, as well as to heal wounds. The lack of some vitamins can have drastic effects. Scurvy, a disease in which wounds heal slowly, gums bleed, and victims become extremely weak, is the result of a severe vitamin C deficiency. This disease was especially common among sailors during the age of wind-powered ships, when weeks or months passed without access to fresh fruits or vegetables. The first clue that a lack of some nutrient was responsible for scurvy came when a Scottish physician named James Lind discovered that eating oranges and lemons could cure the disease. Lind also found that lemon or lime juice could keep scurvy at bay, and he convinced the British Royal Navy to provide a daily ration of juice to its sailors starting in 1795. American sailors found a different cure for the disease: vitamin-C-rich cranberries.

One of the best-known advocates of the healing power of vitamins was Dr. Linus Pauling, an American chemist who won the 1954 Nobel Prize in chemistry and the 1962 Nobel Peace Prize. Though he won his 1954 prize for his analysis of how atoms bond to form chemical compounds, Pauling later examined how vitamins, particularly vitamin C, affected the health of the human body. He believed that huge amounts of vitamin C, which he called *megadoses*, could help people treat ailments such as the common cold and cancer. Indeed, scientists who followed up on Pauling's theories showed that large doses of both vitamin C and vitamin A seemed to prevent some forms of cancer. However, other studies either failed to show any benefit from taking megadoses of vitamins or provided inconclusive results.

Similar studies have yielded similar results regarding the disease-preventing abilities of some minerals, particularly zinc. Minerals are chemical elements such as zinc, calcium, iron, and iodine that the body uses for such functions as building bones, making blood cells, and regulating metabolism. Diets that contain too little or too much of one or more minerals can cause a variety of illnesses. Too little iodine, for instance, causes the thyroid gland to swell to many times its normal size, creating a condition called a *goiter*.

Like vitamins, some minerals have been touted as being able to prevent or cure some illnesses. Perhaps the best-known of these medicinal minerals is zinc, a metal that supposedly can suppress the activity of viruses that cause the common cold or sinus infections. Over the years, zinc has appeared in many products designed to increase the amount of the metal present in the body: tablets, chewing gum, nasal sprays, and health and energy drinks. Despite its popular reputation, though, there have not been many studies analyzing the actual health benefits of zinc supplements and remedies. The few studies that have been conducted have returned varying results, leaving the important question—does the stuff work?—unanswered so far.

Pharmaceutical Foods

Another option is to grow the drugs that people need—not in a laboratory or a factory, but on a farm. Just as genetic engineering techniques make bacteria that can produce insulin, splicing the correct DNA sequence into plants could yield a crop of vegetables that might deliver immunizations, antibiotics, or hormones. Imagine eating a salad made up of lettuce that cures heart disease, tomatoes that prevent influenza, onions that ward off sinus infections, and carrots that reduce tooth decay. Though a meal like this seems unbelievable, scientists are looking into ways to create it.

In fact, such a pharmaceutical salad is not an impossible concept to bring into reality. Botanists already have genetically engineered crop plants such as corn and tomatoes to fight off insects without insecticides, to survive low temperatures in the fields, and to last longer in grocery stores. Scientists have accomplished these feats by splicing in bits of other plants' DNA, creating a genetic *hybrid*. Hybridization is nothing new; such gene-swapping happens naturally between plants that have similar genetics. Farmers performed similar tasks for thousands of years by cross-pollinating different strains to get bigger, hardier, and more nutritious crops. The main difference is that modern-day *transgenic* plants have been created in a laboratory, rather than solely in the fields.

Growing food plants that contain pharmaceutical chemicals could be as simple a job as turning bacteria into insulin factories. The biggest hurdle to overcome is making pharmaceutical food as safe and as reliable as factory-produced drugs. Beyond that hurdle, though, is a bigger political obstacle. People around the world distrust the few *genetically modified*, or GM, crops that already are in production, such as frost-resistant tomatoes. So deep is this distrust that these people often refer to GM crops as *Frankenfoods*, comparing them to the fictional monster that Dr. Frankenstein created out of body parts. For pharmaceutical foods to avoid similar problems, people will have to feel confident that eating such crops will not cause ailments that are worse than the ones being treated or prevented.

14

HERBALISTS AND SCIENTISTS

Herbal medicines and supplements, herb-based teas and cough drops, tinctures combining many natural ingredients that supposedly improve health—the companies that make these compounds and the businesses that sell them have grown into an industry that earns billions of dollars every year. Some of their customers rely on these products as an alternative to the pharmaceuticals of standard Western medicine. Other people incorporate herbs, vitamins, and minerals into their everyday diet in hopes of establishing a barrier against ill health. Decades ago, the only place to find herbal products, aside from supermarket produce sections and spice shelves, was in specialty health-food stores and vitamin shops. Today, a huge assortment of herbs, extracts, and natural additives is for sale virtually anywhere, from coffee shops to convenience stores.

There are, it seems, more supplements and herbal remedies on the market than there are types of OTC medicines. Despite the huge array of manufacturers and brand names, the majority of OTCs fall into just a few classes of drugs (analgesics, antihistamines, diarrhea medicines, and so forth) and specific compounds. A shelf of nonprescription drugs in a pharmacy or a supermarket may, at first, seem like a dramatic array of different drugs in brightly colored boxes. The active ingredients listed on these boxes, though, reveal a fairly limited assortment of chemicals, either working by themselves or combined in multiple-symptom medications. The supplements and remedies of alternative medicine follow a similar pattern, with dozens of manufacturers marketing their own brands of an herbal extract. But there are many more different types of these products than there are of the OTCs, owing to

136

the large number of herbs that people have used for their healing properties over the years.

Then again, new combinations of herbs, vitamins, and the rest of the array of commonly used supplements continually appear on the market, selling in locations ranging from drugstores to commercial sites on the World Wide Web. Radio and television stations constantly run ads for natural aids that, they claim, will help treat afflictions ranging from baldness to bad vision. Some companies even have sold products that supposedly counteract the effects of aging in family pets. Why are there so many of these pills and tablets, these sprays, and elixirs, on the market when OTC drugs have such a narrow range of ingredients? Because the pills, tablets, sprays, and elixirs are not legally considered drugs. Describing them as supplements is not merely a convenient way to refer to them; it is the law.

Under the various safe-food and -drug laws that nations have passed over the years, particularly in the United States, herbs and other botanical products are classified as dietary supplements to indicate that they are not designed to treat illnesses or other medical conditions. At first, vitamins and minerals were the only supplements that really attracted public interest. People need these chemicals in order to live, and they usually can get all they need simply by eating a well-balanced, healthy diet. Physicians and scientists knew for centuries that various foods contained unique nutritional elements that the body required to live. However, the world did not know of vitamins as vitamins until the 1920s, when scientists finally began isolating them from the foods in which they formed.

Classifying vitamins—and minerals, when their importance became known—as dietary supplements reflected their vital role in maintaining normal health, as opposed to the role of pharmaceuticals in attacking microbes or symptoms of illness. Since people needed these chemicals, supplements were freed from having to meet all of the standards that applied to prescription or OTC drugs. All that supplement manufacturers had to do was ensure that their products met the same safety standards that prepared food had to meet, and, later, include nutritional information and warning labels on their packaging. Except in very rare cases, dietary supplements or additives are not seen as things that pose as great a risk of physical damage or overdose as pharmaceuticals do.

Herbs fell under guidelines for dietary supplements, not pharmaceuticals or OTC drugs, because they were derived as extracts of ordinary plants and were not proven to attack any microbe or any biochemical imbalance directly. True, people frequently bought and took herbal supplements intending to use them in place of standard drugs. Manufacturers, though, had to package and market supplements as simple nutritional substances that might aid the body's natural defenses, and not as substances that were designed to treat or cure any disease. This language kept manufacturers from running afoul of enforcement agencies such as the FDA and the U.S. *Federal Trade Commission* (FTC), both of which monitor how food and drug companies present and promote their products.

Today, any combination of herbs, vitamins, minerals, and a few other chemicals can be patented, or at least have its trade name copyrighted, and then go out on the market. Because these products are supplements, they did not have to go through the same multistage testing as pharmaceuticals. At first glance, such supplements might seem to be in the same category as the patent medicines of the past, but there were significant differences. For one thing, the safety requirement means that supplements cannot contain any addictive ingredients such as alcohol or opium. Even the fillers that hold the active ingredients together in pill form or the liquids that make them easier to swallow are chosen both to break down easily in the stomach and to have little or no effect on the body. And all these ingredients, active and inert alike, have to be listed on each supplement's packaging.

The biggest difference between supplements and patent medicines, though, is that herbal and other supplements actually seem to benefit the people who take them. Starting in the early 1990s, there has been a steady increase in the number of people who use dietary supplements either with or in place of standard pharmaceuticals. Herbalists, nutritionists, and physicians who specialize in alternative medical treatments have touted them as safe alternatives to prescription and OTC drugs, which some people consider unsafe. At the same time, some of these supplements seem to be able to treat conditions that standard drugs cannot.

Echinacea and the Common Cold

"If science is so great, why can't it cure the common cold?" This question and ones much like it have been asked repeatedly over the years to point out the limitations of science, that it cannot be expected to solve all the world's problems. The common cold is an especially good example to use, since even today's advances in medicine are not up to the task of curing or preventing this common ailment. Colds are infections of the respiratory system, caused when the mucous membranes come under attack from at least one of more than 100 different types of viruses. The stuffy noses, coughs, fevers, aches, and sore throats that people suffer through are the body's reaction to these viruses, as the microbes hijack the respiratory system and turn it into a virus-making machine. Though most colds last only a few days, some of the most serious cases can develop into lung diseases such as *bronchitis* or *pneumonia*.

A host of products, most of them OTC medications, are available to treat the symptoms of colds, but there is no cure for the cold itself. In order to cure a disease, a drug has to work specifically against the microbes that cause that disease. Antibiotics work by breaking apart the structure of bacteria or interfering with their ability to reproduce. Antiviral drugs, though, work by breaking through the protein shells that viruses build around themselves to survive within the body's hostile environment. To work against viruses, antivirals have to be so powerful that they can kill off beneficial microbes and even healthy body cells. Any drug that could fight each of the viruses that cause the cold probably would create side effects that are worse than the illness they would cure.

Likewise, there are no vaccines for the cold. With so many viruses that cause the common cold, creating a weakened or dead version of each one for use in an anticold shot would be impractical. Even worse, the viruses that cause the common cold evolve rapidly, creating many new strains every year. Keeping up with all of these yearly variations would be impossible. Remember, it takes the better part of a year to analyze the dominant strains of influenza and figure out which three are the most likely to cause problems. Only then is it possible to develop the shot that will help people avoid getting ill during the flu season. Even then, there is no guarantee that the shot will protect against the year's most serious strain—which sometimes turns out to be one that was not expected to show up.

Long before the presence of vaccines and antivirals, though, people turned to teas and poultices made of herbs and other plants to fight off illnesses. One of these healing plants was the purple coneflower, *Echinacea purpurea*, a North American relative of the daisy, which has served for centuries as a remedy for people with weakened immune systems. It does not have the same level of effect as headache-curing willow bark or malaria's natural enemy, the cinchona. When brewed in a tea, though, it seemed to help people who fell ill return to health a bit more quickly. In the last few decades of the 20th century, medical scientists decided to find out exactly what chemicals were responsible for helping the body keep itself feeling better.

Unlike other botanical medicines, echinacea was not as easy for researchers to isolate as was, for example, the chemical salicylate,

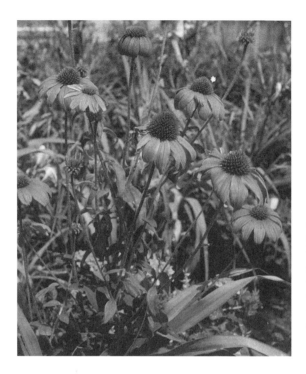

One of the more popular herbal supplement in recent years has been echinacea, which many people believe helps ward off the common cold or shorten the length of its infection. (Larry Allain, United States Geological Survey)

whose discovery led to the creation of aspirin. Even so, herbalists found ways to extract and concentrate whatever chemicals were in the flowers by cooking them and mixing the broth with inert ingredients. Researchers, including physicians and chemists, tested these echinacea extracts on patients and on people who volunteered to help find out what the long-term effects of taking them would be. The results of these experiments seemed to show that something in the flower was doing some good: Patients who took these herbal pills either stayed healthier or recovered from illnesses more rapidly than members of *control groups* who did not take the extracts.

Though not the same as full-fledged pharmaceutical testing, the experiments conducted on the effects of echinacea, and of other botanicals, led to further interest in the subject of herbal medications. Some of this interest showed itself in more detailed tests of the herbs' effects, as well as continued attempts to isolate the chemicals that were having the perceived effect on the immune system. Over the next decade, many of the scientists who conducted this research, as well as herbalists who had known of the herb's healing properties, promoted the benefits of echinacea in books, through magazine articles, and, by the mid-1990s, over the Internet. (These are common forums for the discussion of new trends in medicine. Next to cookbooks, books on medical topics are among every year's best-sellers. Likewise, people always give extra attention to news and feature articles on medical topics.)

At the same time, manufacturers began producing herbal supplements containing echinacea and other herbs, either by themselves or in combination with each other. Goldenseal, another possible immune system booster shown to contain a number of antibiotic chemicals, and ginkgo biloba, which supposedly aided the brain's ability to retain and recall information, joined echinacea to become three of the best-known herbal supplements on the market. Others soon followed. Saint-John's-wort, a shrub with yellow flowers, was promoted as a natural antidepressant, having been used by Europeans for centuries as a calming agent and mood lifter. Even ginger, which cooks around the world use for flavoring, became known as a natural antinausea and motion sickness treatment.

The renewed status of herbs as healing plants, rather than as food ingredients or garden decorations, spread steadily throughout the world. Over time—a fairly short time—people began reading about how well herbal remedies seemed to work and telling each other how much better they felt after taking one of the herb supplements recommended in those books and magazines. They soon knew as much, if not more, about the ancient knowledge of the herbalist than they did of modern medical science. And that was a problem, considering that few people, if any, really know exactly how herbs work.

Proving Herbs Work

The science of herbs, and of alternative medicine in general, has lagged behind its popularity. Like any other field of scientific study, pharmacology operates according to a process of analyzing the physical world in a logical, methodical way. This *scientific method* ensures that the results of a particular study or experiment reflect what actually takes place in the real world, rather than what a researcher would like to believe happens. The scientific method usually falls into five stages: observation, analysis, experimentation, conclusion, and repetition. The observation and analysis phases set the stage for a particular study, when the researcher either observes a natural phenomenon or reviews previous studies that other scientists have conducted, then tries either to explain the phenomenon or to find potential sources of error in previous studies. Experimentation is the stage in which the researcher puts his or her analysis to the test, seeking either to confirm that an explanation is correct or to discover why it is not. The conclusion and repetition stages are when the researcher determines what the results of his or her experiments mean and makes sure that the initial experiment was not itself in error.

The scientific method is not perfect—as the world's experience with thalidomide in the 1960s showed—but it has proven itself over time to be the most reliable method for determining the reasons behind physical phenomena. Within the experimentation phase is the concept of the control-group study, in which a group being studied is compared to a group that, basically, is ignored during the study, except for occasional monitoring. Control groups are a way to verify that, in the case of pharmaceutical research, a particular drug is responsible for a set of changes: If both groups undergo similar changes, than the drug likely is not the reason for the change. The procedure for approving new drugs, with its multiple laboratory and clinical testing phases, uses expanded versions of this control-group study method.

However, most of the news about the effects of herbal medication in the mid-to-late 1990s consisted of stories of people who said they felt better after taking herbs and other extracts for their health. This type of information, which is based on how people describe their own feelings and reactions, is called *anecdotal evidence*. While anecdotes can point out areas of study that need to be explored, anecdotes themselves are not science. They cannot be confirmed experimentally, because every person's perceptions are different. Anecdotes also can be false. Not only can unscrupulous researchers and marketers make up stories about a supplement's healing powers (as happened during the days of the medicine show), but also people can succumb to the *placebo effect:* They will feel better because they have been told that a pill will *make* them feel better.

Until the mid-to-late 1990s, almost no one in the Western world had subjected herbal medicines to the same scrutiny given to pharmaceuticals. The few tests that had been conducted were done in laboratories or in nonclinical tests. In Asia and Africa, herbal medicines were a part of health care that had been in existence for thousands of years. Few people saw the need to analyze these time-tested remedies. In the meantime, companies in Europe and North America added herbal extracts to everyday products, from skin moisturizers to sodas and "energy drinks." None of these products promised to cure any particular ailment or to create any specific improvement in health, mainly because doing so was illegal. Instead, their manufacturers marketed these products as contributing to an allover beneficial effect by enhancing the body's natural chemistry.

The popularity of herbs and the widespread use of herbal extracts finally led university and government researchers to begin scientific studies of whether herbal medicines actually work and how they interact with the body and with other drugs. Chemists began analyzing the chemical makeup of these plants in greater detail than they had before, while microbiologists started gauging their effects against microbes in the same way that antibiotic molds had been tested decades before. Private and public medical research institutions took part in this research, most of them working as part of a government-sponsored program to test the safety of herbal supplements as well as the health claims of alternative-medicine advocates.

A Pharmaceutical Look at Herbs

So, what have these studies revealed about the healing power of herbs so far? Unfortunately, not much. The researchers had a lot of catching up to do at the beginning of the 21st century. Much of their early work involved building a base of knowledge about alternative medicine that had been established for scientific medicine more than a century before. Despite the widespread use of herbal supplements and a large number of health care professionals who specialized in alternative medicinal methods, there was little hard science to start with. Thus far, this work has not been going on long enough for evidence to prove or disprove the effects of herbal extracts.

Given that there was a lot of work to do, these projects did yield some interesting results early on, though these findings were not always favorable to the proponents of herbal remedies. Some studies of Saint-John's-wort, which had been lauded as a natural antidepressant, showed it to be no more effective than a placebo when treating severe forms of depression. Others, though, showed that the herb indeed lifted the mood of people with milder cases, and to a degree that could not be explained as simply the result of a placebo effect. Other studies confirmed the presence of disease-fighting compounds in such plants as garlic, goldenseal, and echinacea, though their actual disease-fighting ability still was questionable.

Proponents of herbal supplements held firm to their reliance on these products. Some accused the researchers of selecting the wrong type of each herb to study. For instance, a number of tests on echinacea indicated that its status as an immune-system booster was overrated, and that the flower only had a slight effect on helping the body ward off or overcome disease. Some critics of these studies said the results came from using a different species of echinacea from *Echinacea purpurea*, which was credited with having the greatest health benefits. Others said that these tests, and tests of different herbs, used extracts and pills that were prepared incorrectly.

Yet another criticism of these early studies was that they were yielding preliminary results, and that future investigations would bear out the value of herbal preparations. Such critiques were accurate, in that one or two studies are not enough to create a full picture of any phenomenon. Even so, the initial results were seen as a dash of cold water that cooled down the furor over herbal products. They were especially timely considering that some negative effects of herbs were coming to light.

15

WARNING SIGNS

Much of the appeal of herbal products comes from the fact that herbs are products of nature, not laboratories. Advertisements for herbal supplements constantly use the word *natural,* conjuring up images of freshly grown ingredients being harvested from gardens, fields, or forest glens before being processed in surroundings that look like brick-oven bakeries or old-time breweries. Of course, modern bakeries and breweries buy their ingredients in huge bulk loads and process them in factories that contain stainless steel piping and automated machinery, rather than wooden kneading boards and oak barrels. The same goes for companies that make herbal products, which can be just as mechanized and profit-driven as the world's largest pharmaceutical firms.

Describing herbal products as "natural" has one important effect, though. It taps into an idea that many people share about other mass-produced supplements and medications: the idea that laboratory-produced chemicals are less effective and less safe than those obtained from natural sources. The body, this belief goes, cannot absorb and use synthetically produced chemicals as efficiently as those from nature. And, although the ads and the labels do not say so directly, there is an implied message that herbal supplements are safer to take than synthetically produced pharmaceuticals precisely because they are natural.

Chemically speaking, such is rarely the case. Provided they have the same molecular structure, nutritional chemicals created in a laboratory are the same as chemicals derived from plants and other natural sources. The body can absorb and use a nutrient, such as a vitamin or a mineral, no matter what its source. True, there are exceptions. A few studies have indicated that the natural forms of some vitamins work better than synthetically produced forms. Allergic reactions to a particular form of nutrient, depending on its source or the ingredients with which it is mixed, also can determine if a natural or a synthetic supplement is safest. People who are allergic to shellfish, for example, are better off avoiding calcium supplements created from oyster shells.

In general, though, the safety of an herbal supplement, like the safety of a pharmaceutical drug, does not depend on the supplement's source as much as it does on the supplement's ingredients. Some herbs can cause heart problems, circulatory system problems, or damage to other organs. Herbs can react badly with prescription or OTC drugs, either weakening their effect or enhancing their power to the point where patients suffer an overdose from an otherwise safe amount of medicine. An herbal product's safety also can depend on the person or company that prepares it. There are no firm standards that say how much of an herb or an herbal extract is enough to create an effect in the body. Even worse, there is no way to determine if an herbal product actually contains the herb or herbs that are listed on its label. Much of the herbal supplement business is based on the honor system, and that system too often seems to break down.

An Herb Clashes with a Drug

Herbs and pharmaceuticals often do not mix well. During the 1990s, a plant called Saint-John's-wort became one of the most widely known and widely used herbs in the United States. A shrub with small green leaves and yellow flowers, Saint-John's-wort seemed to be a safe, natural substitute for many pharmaceutical antidepressants. For centuries, the story went, Europeans drank herbal teas made of Saint-John's-wort to combat mild cases of depression, especially in northern Europe, where winter nights last longer than they do farther south. Many people in these regions develop a form of depression called *seasonal affective disorder* (SAD), which is also called winter depression or winter blues. SAD comes from the decrease in sunlight as the days shorten between mid-fall and early spring, and its symptoms are similar to those of other depressive maladies.

Depression, in psychiatric terms, is not an overbearing feeling of sadness. Instead, it refers to a depressed flow of electrochemical signals through the neurons of the brain caused by a reduction in neurochem-

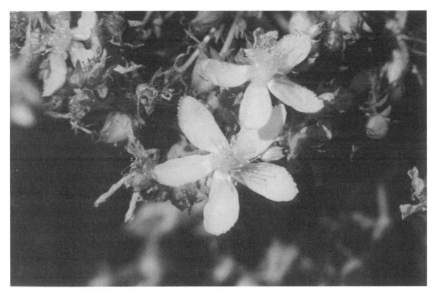

Saint-John's-wort, an herb that some people take as a natural antidepressant, has been shown to cause problems when taken in combination with certain pharmaceutical drugs. [National Plant Data Center/plants.usda.gov]

icals such as serotonin and dopamine. Symptoms of this neurochemical shortage include sleeplessness, difficulty thinking, mood swings, as well as emotional lows. Through chemical reactions inside and between the neurons, antidepressants keep the levels of brain chemicals "normal." From the end of World War II on, psychiatric researchers discovered a wide selection of prescription antidepressants, many of which are described in Chapter 7. These drugs shared the ability to speed up and strengthen the flow of signals through the brain, though at the cost of some annoying side effects.

Saint-John's-wort supposedly was able to combat depression without the side effects of psychiatric drugs, and some people with depression began using the herb instead of, or along with, standard antidepressant medications. Many of the people who used the herb instead of the medications did so because they distrusted pharmaceuticals and Western medicine in general, or because of a desire to live a "more natural" lifestyle. Others were not able to afford psychiatric care and medication, and turned to Saint-John's-wort as an affordable alternative. Some patients who were under psychiatric care and were taking antidepressant medications used Saint-John's-wort as well, believing that the herbal supplement would not affect or interfere with their prescribed medications. Most of these people, studies showed, did not tell their psychiatrists or their physicians about their supplemental self-medication.

Without realizing it, these patients were putting themselves at great risk of developing additional problems, perhaps worse than the ones they were trying to treat. Overcoming depression with medicine is a chemical balancing act. Patients have to have a high enough level of antidepressant drugs in their bloodstream to overcome the *blood-brain barrier*, which prevents foreign substances from entering the brain. Too little of a drug in the patient's bloodstream and there will be no effect; however, too much of a drug can numb a patient to reality, while also threatening to damage the liver, the kidneys, and other organs.

For all of its image as a centuries-old cure from nature, Saint-John's-wort contains a mix of chemical compounds that supposedly do the same thing as pharmaceutical antidepressants. When patients began taking the herb along with prescribed antidepressants, the chemicals from the two sources enhanced each other, causing a greater reaction in the patients' brains. Some patients began showing up with signs of antidepressant overdose, although they were taking well-adjusted doses of antidepressants. In rare cases, Saint-John's-wort even counteracted some pharmaceutical antidepressants, leaving patients feeling as bad as they did before. Even worse was the interaction between Saint-John's-wort and a class of drugs called protease inhibitors, which help prevent infections of human immunodeficiency virus (HIV) from developing into AIDS. A number of studies showed that the herb cut down the amount of the HIV-suppressing drug that was present in the bloodstream, putting patients at greater risk of developing the disease. Since many HIV patients naturally felt depressed about their condition and the stress it put on them, some of them were taking Saint-John's-wort without knowing the possible harm they were doing to themselves.

There was, it turned out, no safe way to combine Saint-John's-wort with any prescribed or OTC medications. As with other herbal products, the amounts of Saint-John's-wort in commercially produced supplements varied widely. No minimum or maximum dosages of the herb or of its active ingredients had been determined as of early 2003, though some studies of the herb's effect used amounts ranging from a few hundred milligrams to a gram and a half a day. Because there was no reliable way to know how much of the herb was too much, manufacturers were asked to include warnings about the plant's possible problems on their product labels, while pharmacists began including warnings about Saint-John's-wort in the literature they gave their customers.

Dangerous Interactions Revisited

Saint-John's-wort is far from being alone in posing great health risks to those who decide to take herbal supplements for their health. Many herbs can react with prescription or OTC drugs to cause such problems as bleeding and organ damage, or the herbs can cancel out the healing properties of the pharmaceutical medicines altogether. Some herbal supplements or remedies can cause serious damage to the body on their own.

For years, people who have trouble losing weight have been able to turn to OTC diet pills or more-powerful prescription medications that cut hunger pangs and cause the body to burn more calories. In the 1990s, though, a different type of weight-loss medication came out. Called fen-phen, it was a combination of two existing prescription diet drugs that already were widely used to combat obesity. The "fen" in the mixture's name came from *fenfluramine* and a related drug called *dexfenfluramine*, either of which was mixed with *phentermine*, which contributed the "phen."

Studies in the early 1990s showed that seriously obese people lost large amounts of weight when they took combinations of the two types of drugs. The drugs had not been approved for use in this combination, but physicians were able to prescribe the drugs under the off-label rules. And while fen-phen did not become available in a single pill, prescriptions for the two drugs soared over the next few years. Fen-phen became one of the most-prescribed medications in the world: In 1996 prescriptions in the United States alone totaled more than 18 million.

However, problems with the combination had begun showing up long before then. In 1994 physicians began noticing that an unusually high number of patients, mostly women in their 30s and 40s, were developing leaky heart valves. Normally, the valves that separate the chambers of the heart from each other and from main *arteries* and *veins* seal completely, forcing blood to flow in just one direction. When the tissue of the valves becomes damaged—from old age, from disease, or from poisoning by foreign chemicals—the valves fail to close completely, allowing some blood to leak backward. This leakage makes a noise called a *heart murmur* that physicians can detect using very sensitive microphones.

Heart-valve damage such as this usually does not occur in people younger than 50 and often is the result of poor health habits. Unless treated, the disorder can lead to more serious problems. Since the damaged valves no longer prevent the blood from moving backward, the heart has to work harder to keep the blood flowing at the proper pressure. Just as driving uphill in low gear can cause a car's engine to overheat and break down, leaky valves can lead to permanent damage to the heart muscle, leaving it unable to pump effectively and resulting in a condition called congestive heart failure.

As the physicians who noticed this premature valve damage examined their patient's medical histories, they discovered that all had developed this problem after they started taking fen-phen. Before long, these physicians had identified more than 100 patients who suffered from heart valve problems that seemed to be associated with fen-phen, and at least 87 more who had abnormal *echocardiograms*, measurements of the sound the heart makes. This was only a tiny fraction of the millions of people who were using fen-phen, but it was enough to worry physicians and regulators alike.

Further studies identified fenfluramine and dexfenfluramine as the agents responsible for the damage. By 1997 a handful of nations around the world, including the United States, banned the two drugs, or at least asked manufacturers to voluntarily remove them from the market. Phentermine was and still is allowed to stay in production, as there was no indication that it was responsible for any serious negative effects. However, the people who had come to rely on the fen-phen combination to aid or maintain their weight loss were unhappy at losing the "fen" drugs, and they began looking for an effective alternative.

When they found one, it turned out to be an herbal preparation called ma huang. Also known as *ephedra*, ma huang is a Chinese herb that contains a chemical called *ephedrine*, which physicians prescribe to combat the symptoms and attacks of asthma. Ephedrine also is chemically similar to a decongestant called *pseudoephedrine*, which is sold in OTC medications and in combination with prescription drugs. Part of ephedrine's ability to combat asthma comes from its ability to stimulate the body's metabolism into working faster, boosting the rate of oxygen transfer in the lungs and its distribution throughout the body. This stimulation also causes the body to convert fat to energy at a greater rate then normal, one that approaches the activity of fenfluramine and dexfenfluramine. Here, then, was the "fen" replacement that dieters had been seeking. Ma huang became the main ingredient in herbal supplements referred to as natural or herbal-based fen-phens.

The manufacturers of this new alternative to fen-phen said their products were safe if used as directed. Within a couple of years, though, physicians and public interest groups began reporting as many deaths from ephedra as from fen-phen. It turned out that, as with many other stimulants, the levels of ephedra in ma huang increased heart rates and boosted blood pressure, putting people at greater risk for heart attacks and strokes. Researchers who specialized in sports medicine said that ephedrine also might be partly to blame for the deaths by heatstroke of 15 professional football players between 1995 and 2001 during preseason training, more than twice as many as those who died from 1985 to 1994. As part of its stimulating effect, ephedrine raises body temperature and reduces sweating, two changes that can be disastrous in athletes who spend their time exercising strenuously outdoors. Add in the fact that the herb also masked the feelings of pain and fatigue that the athletes felt during their workouts, and ephedra was clearly an herb that was too dangerous to use.

Football players wanted to use ephedra precisely because the herb was a short-term energy booster, one that could give them an edge over opposing players during a game. But the dangers that the drug posed to the athletes' health, and the desire to prevent athletes from using drugs to achieve an advantage over their opponents, led both the National Football League and the National Collegiate Athletic Association to ban ephedrine and pseudoephedrine, which caused many of the same effects as ephedrine. Many other groups have asked that these products be banned in general, or at least banned from nonprescription uses. In the United States, the FDA ruled in 2002 that it needed more information on ephedra's effects before deciding whether or not to prohibit its use altogether.

Quality Control

One of the biggest obstacles to determining the danger or safety of herbal supplements is the wide variation in the quality and quantity of herbs and nonherbal ingredients that go into these compounds. Supplements are generally unsupervised by the government. Manufacturers are responsible for making sure that their products are safe and for not making any claims that they can treat specific maladies. The same goes for car manufacturers being responsible for making sure their products are safe to drive and for not encouraging their customers to enter stock-car races or drive up the sides of canyons. Any policing of supplement makers comes after their products reach the market and begin to have an effect on consumers.

As of early 2003 there was no way to guarantee that any herbal supplement contained exactly what its label proclaimed. As with the patent medicines of the 19th century, any herbal product could contain all,

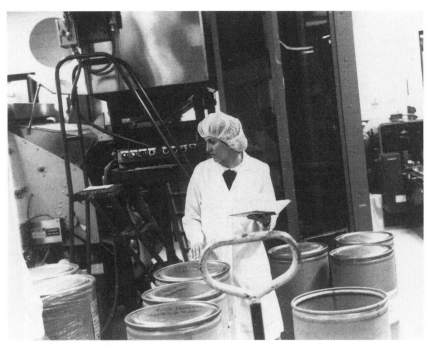

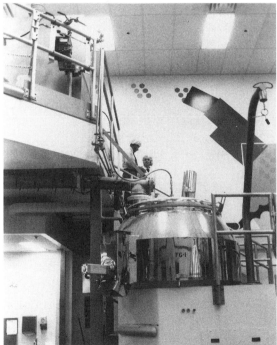

Each year, FDA investigators inspect thousands of pharmaceutical companies. In these photographs an investigator checks bulk containers of raw materials and examines part of the manufacturing process to make sure the equipment is functioning properly. (Courtesy Food and Drug Administration)

some, or none of the promised active ingredient or extract. One manufacturer's echinacea tablet, for instance, could contain 500 milligrams of the herb while another could contain 750 milligrams of an extract of the herb. Since there was no such thing as a standard effective dose of echinacea, the average consumer could not judge which tablet was the right one to take. Unless they got advice from a knowledgeable physician, a pharmacist, or a local herbalist, or read a number of books on herbs and herbal lore, consumers who wanted to see if herbal supplements were right for them basically had to experiment on themselves.

A related problem affected both herbal supplements and herbal "medicines" prepared by independent herbalists as part of the alternative medicine movement. There have been many cases over the years of herbal supplements and independently produced herbal preparations that contain banned prescription drugs or nonprescription ingredients. In one case in Britain, an herbalist mixed batches of weight-loss pills that contained fenfluramine as well as herbal ingredients. Customers were not told about this addition, only that the products were "safe" and "natural." The herbalist probably ordered the fenfluramine from an overseas manufacturer and was able to sneak it past Britain's customs inspectors, as countries that ban the drug are vastly outnumbered by those that do not. Other cases of deliberate deception have included herbal remedies that include such dangerous elements as mercury and lead.

As part of research into herbs and herbal remedies, scientists and governmental agencies are determining how to regulate these products. The question is whether to treat herbs as OTC drugs, as prescription drugs, or as simple dietary supplements (the way they are now). Manufacturers, herbalists, and some physicians want to have matters left to public choice. Ultimately, the answer probably will come as the result of the same analysis that is used for determining the safety and efficacy of pharmaceuticals.

PART 5

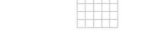

Resistance Movements

16

DRUG-RESISTANT GERMS

There are good reasons to investigate the pharmaceutical uses of herbs and herbal medicines, despite the dangers. The modern medicines that once seemed likely to turn infectious diseases into little more than a bad memory have begun to lose their power over their deadly foes. The problem is not that the drugs are less potent, but that the microbes they fought have reemerged in new, tougher forms. These germs are returning to plague humanity just as they did long ago, and medical science is racing to hold them back.

Trouble in the Hospital

Hospitals always have been places where people risk picking up an infection. As an inevitable side effect of having large numbers of ill or injured people in such a confined area, disease microbes travel from host to host and establish colonies within any machinery that allows them to live and multiply. Even in the largest medical centers with the most sophisticated filtering systems and sanitation procedures, a lot of time and effort goes to preventing and combating infections.

The disinfectants that perfume hospital corridors and rooms hold down the microbes that can be deposited by a patient's sneeze or along with a fingerprint. Though bacterial infections can spring up in patients following surgery, antibiotics have been able to keep them in check. But it is not possible to eliminate all the infectious disease microbes within a hospital building. Physicians and nurses travel from

DEVELOPING DRUG RESISTANCE IN THE HOSPITAL

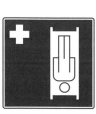

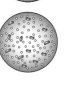

1) Patients with different maladies enter a hospital. The enclosed conditions provide a perfect place for germs to spread, even with rigorous sanitation and disease control practices.

2) Hospital staff administers standard antibiotics and other antimicrobial drugs both to patients who come in sick and to patients who pick up diseases after arriving.

3) Over time, microbes such as bacteria and viruses evolve an immunity to the most commonly prescribed drugs.

4) The drug-resistant microbes work their way into the hospital population, infecting patients, visitors, and health care workers. Not everyone will come down with a resistant disease, but some will act as carriers.

5) As more patients fall ill to drug-resistant diseases, physicians have to turn to more powerful drugs. Over time the process repeats until, some people fear, it reaches the point where there are no drugs left to fight one or more diseases.

Unfortunately, despite the good they do, hospitals also can serve as points for the incubation and spread of disease. This diagram shows how an infection can strengthen and spread in a hospital.

patient to patient at all hours, and new patients arrive with new diseases all the time. Patients die from postoperative infections or from diseases such as pneumonia that they contract during their stay. A late-1990s estimate showed that of the 2 million or so hospital patients who come down with an infection during their stay, about 5 percent—90,000 people—succumb to the new disease. But these deaths, though tragic, are not unexpected, and modern hospitals usually have been able to keep these diseases under control. That is, unless the microbes manage to outwit the medicines.

Almost as soon as World War II ended, people began benefiting from the sudden flood of antibiotics that followed the penicillin revolution. Vaccination, antiviral drugs, and drugs to combat parasitic infections played equally effective roles in raising lifespans and expectations of good health. Hidden among these medical success stories, though, were signs of trouble for the future. During his experiments with penicillin, Sir Alexander Fleming noticed that some *Staphylococcus* bacteria seemed to adapt to and live with the drug. Before the end of the 1940s, hospitals around the world experienced outbreaks of bacterial infections that seemed to ignore some antibiotics. Such resistance to the effects of penicillin, streptomycin, and similar drugs was unusual, however, and the public neither noticed nor seemed to care about the wonder drugs' sudden vulnerability.

During the next two decades, microbes and medicine ran a close race to see which side would dominate the other. For the most part, healing drugs kept ahead of diseases. Then, things began tipping in the microbes' favor. Two types of bacteria—*Haemophilus influenzae*, which causes some respiratory infections, and *Neisseria gonorrhaeae*, the source of the venereal disease gonorrhea—developed strains that essentially ate penicillin in the mid-1970s. With both bacteria, the invulnerable strain appeared in people who were taking penicillin as a way to prevent disease, rather than to cure it. The resistant *gonorrhaeae*, in particular, developed during the Vietnam War in South Vietnamese prostitutes who were taking penicillin precisely to avoid coming down with gonorrhea.

As with earlier drug-resistant germs, physicians were able to treat these strains with stronger antibiotics or with drugs that boosted the immune system. However, using more powerful drugs created other problems. Antibiotics do not just target microbes that cause disease. Once the drugs reach the bloodstream, they can kill any bacterium in their path, even ones that have no effect on the body. These bugs do a valuable service for the people they inhabit: by taking up space in the body, they deny diseases a place to grow. Eliminating these harmless germs opens up living space for harmful microbes. Other bacteria, such as *Escherichia coli*, aid digestion, and killing them off wreaks havoc in the intestines until new *E. coli* move in.

Using more powerful antibiotics also leads to the development of more powerful germs. For the rest of the 1970s and throughout the 1980s, hospitals and physicians reported that previously simple infections were resisting standard drugs. Soon, bacteria began developing the ability to fight off a spectrum of progressively stronger drugs. Microbiologists created a new term to describe these bacteria, as well as other microbes that were becoming immune to many medicines: the *multiple-drug-resistant*, or MDR, microbe. MDR bacteria are the most common of this new class of microbes. They are the ones that resist most antibiotics except for drugs such as vancomycin, which is so potent that it has been used as a "drug of last resort." One of the greatest public-health fears is that a widespread vancomycin-resistant disease might appear one day.

Old Enemies Return

The real threat of MDR microbes is not simply the ability to shrug off antibiotics that once defeated them. The truly alarming fact is that such resistance is bringing back microbes and diseases that people thought had been tamed. Foremost among these germs are the *Staphylococcus* and *Streptococcus* bacteria that cause health problems such as sore throats, skin infections, and eye diseases. Ironically, these two types of bacteria were precisely the ones that penicillin first was mass-produced to defeat. Fleming's discovery of penicillin came from a culture of *Staphylococcus aureus* he had been studying. The drug's first partial victory was a patient who developed a combined *Staphylococcus* and *Streptococcus* infection, and who died only because there was not enough of the drug to continue his near-miraculous recovery.

These days, strains of *Streptococcus* and *Staphylococcus* have evolved shields against penicillin and stronger antibiotics, much as a rhinoceros evolved its thick hide to protect against predator attacks. Worse, these long-standing bacterial foes are developing new ways to infect people. One of the most notorious of these illnesses is *necrotizing fasciitis*, nicknamed the "flesh-eating disease" because it kills and devours healthy skin cells. The culprit behind this disease is a formerly mild *Streptococcus* bacterium, such as those that live on the skin and do little more than cause boils (unless they get inside the body through a scratch or a cut). In its more powerful form, this bacterium can attack people whose immune systems have been weakened by other illnesses, as well as some healthy people who have the misfortune to come across it.

Far worse diseases have made more dramatic comebacks, thanks to their drug resistance. Tuberculosis, the lung infection caused by the *Mycobacterium tuberculosis* bacteria, long held sway as one of the deadly consequences of urban life. An airborne bacterium, *M. tuberculosis* nestles in the lungs after being coughed or sneezed out by someone who suffers from the disease. Crowded city conditions make it easy for tuberculosis to jump from person to person, especially people arriving who lack immunity to the diseases of the city. From the late 18th to the early 20th century, tuberculosis—also called *TB* or *consumption* because it seemed to slowly devour its victims—was one of many maladies that struck city dwellers either in periodic outbreaks or in ongoing epidemics. The arrival of antibiotics drastically cut down the number of tuberculosis cases in the developed world, though it remained a problem in prisons and in poorer nations.

With the arrival of the 1990s came disturbing reports of new tuberculosis strains. Most of these cases appeared in the developing world, which consists mainly of nations in Africa, South America, and Southeast Asia. Poverty, poor sanitation, and substandard health care in these countries, combined with unreliable supplies of medicine, helped drug-resistant TB bacteria to emerge. The developed world was not immune, however. A major epidemic of tuberculosis broke out in New York City in the late 1980s and early 1990s, starting in the city's vast jail system and spreading to hospitals and the public. Nineteen ninety-two was the worst year. More than 3,800 cases of TB, 441 of them involving multiple-drug-resistant strains, broke out. Hundreds of people died from both the conventional and the MDR strains, though most of the deaths involved patients who also have been battling HIV infections or AIDS. This double whammy of disease, in fact, was one of the reasons why the MDR strains developed. Many of the New York prisoners were taking a combination of drugs to supplement their weakened immune systems. It was only natural that some TB bacteria would evolve into a superstrain.

Fortunately, New York City and state health officials were able to halt the epidemic by closely monitoring TB patients and using a regimen of very powerful antibiotics. However, this outbreak and others that have taken place elsewhere across the globe show how vulnerable the world is to serious diseases, even ones that people thought were defeated.

But how can microbes develop resistance to antibiotics or other medicines? First, drugs rarely kill every microbe within a patient. There always will be a small percentage of organisms that naturally are immune to a particular drug. The goal is to wipe out enough microbes for the immune system to gain an advantage over the rest. In some cases, random *mutations*, or changes in the genetic code, of a microbe will give it the ability to survive exposure to a drug. In other cases, a drug will be weak enough for strong microbes to survive and pass on their traits both to their offspring and to other microbes. At times, the microbe that provides the resistant traits does not have to be related to the microbe that received them. All that is needed is the transfer of the right segment of DNA from one to another.

Bacteria in particular trade drug resistance like baseball cards. Some bacteria transfer DNA through *conjugation*, an extremely primitive sexual process of transmitting chemical information through a long *flagellum*, or chemical thread, running from a donor to a recipient. Other bacteria pick up DNA sequences by consuming different bacterial strains, either living ones that succumb to predatory germs or dead ones that died from some cause other than a particular antibiotic. Even viruses can transmit the chemical codes that provide antibiotic resistance—the average bacteria is more than 10 times as large as the largest virus, and many viruses have evolved to reproduce within bacteria. In the process, the viruses pick up genetic sequences from the bacteria, incorporate it into their own genetic code, and then pass it on to other bacteria.

By hijacking genetic codes from the cells they invade, viruses also have adapted themselves to ward off the effects of antiviral drugs and some of the more powerful antibiotics. A virus is little more than a chain of genetic code, either DNA or RNA, protected in a shell of protein molecules. By itself, a virus is not alive: It does not eat, reproduce, move about under its own power, or even seek out cells it can infect. A virus only becomes active when it brushes up against a living cell whose walls contain the right *receptors*, chemicals that fit the structure of the virus and allow it to open a passage to the cell's interior. Once inside, the viral DNA or RNA makes its way into the cell's nucleus, taking over its normal genetic code and turning the cell into a virus factory. When this process begins, the cell begins producing viruses that combine the parent's genetic code with any sequences that make the jump from the cell's DNA to the virus. If the sequences help the new viruses live long enough to find their own host cells, those traits will find their way into future generations; if not, the viruses will die out.

Fungi and parasites use similar methods to improve their ability to survive and reproduce. All these microbes, though, likely would not be modifying themselves as rapidly as they have been if it were not for the medicines that force them to evolve. Nor is it just the drugs that have led to the creation of resistant strains.

Giving Drugs a Rest

In war, an army's least enviable job is to retake ground it once occupied but lost to a stronger and retrenched foe. The job becomes even worse when the enemy regains the contested ground not as the result of a particularly brilliant strategy but simply by capitalizing on the once-victorious army's mistakes. Modern medical scientists are in just this position with the resurgence of old diseases in drug-resistant forms, and they now find themselves scrambling to regain the edge that medicine once had over the microbes.

Without meaning to, humans have been helping disease germs in their fight to resist the effects of modern pharmaceuticals. The rise of resistant bacteria offers a typical example of how people have contributed to the problems of drug resistance. For decades, people who come down with viral infections from influenza to the common cold have cajoled their physicians into prescribing penicillin or another antibiotic to treat their illness. The problem is that, with very few exceptions, antibiotics have never been able to harm viruses. Most antibiotics work in one of three ways: They attack a cell's wall, opening holes in the protective barrier and exposing the interior to the elements; they interrupt the cell's reproductive process; or they travel inside the cell and disrupt its metabolism. The problem with viruses, of course, is that viruses are not cells. Until a virus attaches itself to an appropriate host cell, it cannot even be considered to be alive. And once a virus infects a host, it is shielded from the effects of antibiotics, which mostly do not react with body cells.

Unfortunately, a lot of patients either do not know about this quirk of antibiotics, or choose not to believe it exists. They will ask a physician to prescribe antibiotics for a viral disease. When told that the drug will do no good, they will argue that they have taken antibiotics for the same condition in the past, they know their symptoms better than the physician does, or they will simply find another doctor who will give them the medicine they want. Physicians often end up giving in to these requests, reasoning that the drugs will combat *opportunistic infections* from bacteria that have been taking advantage of their patients' weakened immune systems. Others simply find it easier to write the prescription than to try to explain why the drugs will not work. Over the years, all these unneeded prescriptions have exposed bacteria to varying amounts of antibiotics, increasing their chances to adapt to the drugs and develop resistant strains.

At the same time, patients have helped bacteria through improper use of antibiotics, whether needed or not. Antibiotic prescriptions are

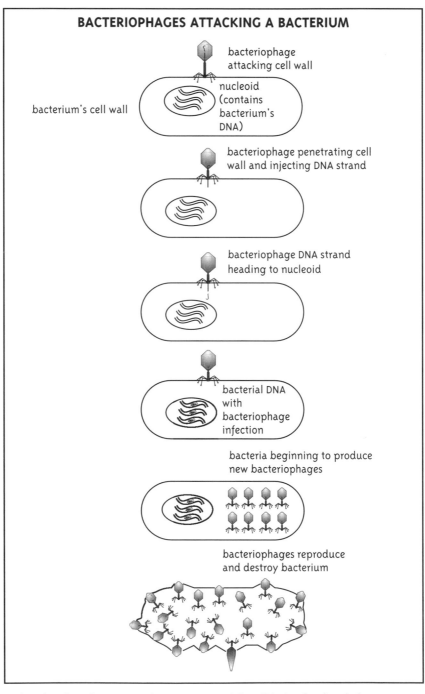

BACTERIOPHAGES ATTACKING A BACTERIUM

bacteriophage
attacking cell wall

nucleoid
(contains
bacterium's
DNA)

bacterium's cell wall

bacteriophage penetrating cell
wall and injecting DNA strand

bacteriophage DNA strand
heading to nucleoid

bacterial DNA
with
bacteriophage
infection

bacteria beginning to produce
new bacteriophages

bacteriophages reproduce
and destroy bacterium

Rather than focusing on creating more powerful antibiotics that break down
bacteria cell walls, some researchers are trying to adapt bacteriophages, viruses
that prey on bacteria, as medical drugs.

designed to give patients a constant amount of the drug that lasts from four days to two weeks—enough time to fight off the infection. Many patients, though, stop taking their prescription a day or two early, thinking that they will save some of the often-pricey antibiotics to treat a later infection. This method, of course, is ideal for filtering out the strongest bacteria and giving them the opportunity to thrive. Even if the patient is fortunate enough not to develop a more serious infection from these invigorated microbes, he or she still can pass them on to other people, possibly starting a new epidemic.

Similar problems arise when treating fungal or parasitic infections with either an inappropriate medicine or with a medicine that a patient stops taking too early. Such misuses are part of the reason behind the separation of prescription and OTC drugs. Most people do not know enough about medicine to determine which prescription drugs will best treat which diseases and which drugs they should avoid. It is up to physicians to decide which drugs to prescribe and to explain to their patients why they should not use other drugs. Fortunately, an increasing number of physicians began taking a firmer stance against writing unnecessary prescriptions in the late 1990s and early 2000s. Government health agencies and professional medical groups also took part in this effort, conducting advertising campaigns to warn people about the dangers of antibiotic misuse and to teach them the difference between bacterial and viral infections. Still, asking for and prescribing antibiotics is a decades-long habit that may take years to break. Until then, there will be patients and physicians who assist microbes in their battle to overcome humanity's modern medical armory.

17

THE PERILS OF MEDICINE

There is no such thing as risk-free medication, whether it comes from a doctor's prescription or the shelves of a drugstore's cough-and-cold aisle. People who use modern medicines responsibly are vulnerable to unpleasant side effects as much as they are to the rise of drug-resistant microbes. When people use pharmaceutical drugs improperly, they make themselves vulnerable to problems that are far worse than the ones they are trying to cure. The risk is even greater if the drugs contain contaminants.

In a way, taking medicine is very much like conducting a *black-box experiment*. This term refers to an attempt to analyze any structure—a cell, an atom, a distant star—without being able to look inside it. Nuclear physics, for example, is based on decades of black-box experiments. It is not yet possible to see the makeup of an atom's electrons, protons, and neutrons directly. Scientists therefore use *particle accelerators* to do the next best thing—launch atoms or subatomic particles into each other at high speeds and analyze the energy tracks of the pieces that fly apart. By mathematically reassembling these fragments, physicists can estimate how the original atoms and particles fit together.

A similar thing happens every time a patient begins taking a new medicine. There is no way to predict exactly how any drug will affect every patient who takes it. The drug's clinical trials can provide a list of side effects that may appear, but such a list can serve only as a guideline. Patients' reactions to the drugs they take are the only clues their physicians have about what is happening inside their bodies.

Unfortunately, pharmaceuticals pose many dangers for the people who take them that go beyond harmful side effects or allergic reactions. Some of the most powerful drugs also can be extremely addictive, chemically wiring the patient's brain or body to depend on them in order to function. Of course, how people normally treat medicine has a lot to do with their vulnerability to addiction. The most fortunate people are the ones who think of medicines as nothing more than a chemical tool to fight disease or counteract pain and injury. If there are any withdrawal symptoms, such as from an antibiotic or a painkiller that the body has become used to, then the best thing is to get over them as quickly as possible. A few people turn to medicines only as a last resort, if at all. Some people avoid pharmaceutical drugs for religious reasons, considering them unnatural and thus not allowed by their beliefs. Others simply dislike the idea of relying on a pill for their health and decide to deal with their maladies as best they can.

Then there are the people who view drugs in the same way that people in ancient times viewed magic: as an unknown but all-powerful force that will cure any physical problem they have. These people place their utter trust in pharmaceuticals, and in the physicians who prescribe them. They are ones who are most likely to turn to medicines immediately when they have a problem, and they are highly likely to become dependent on their drugs.

On the other side of the pharmacy counter, there is the danger of either accidental or deliberate contamination of drugs. Such types of tampering have caused serious health crises around the world, including cases of poisoning that many people have considered the equivalent of terrorism campaigns. The safety seals, tamper-resistant packaging, and similar features of modern drug packaging came about to counteract these threats, and in large part they have succeeded. They have not been foolproof, though, and many patients have suffered because someone found a way around these safeguards.

One other danger lies in the easy ways people can get drugs. Many legitimate medicines are highly addictive and have side effects that appeal to people searching for pharmaceutical intoxication. Although they are tightly regulated, narcotic prescription painkillers can become recreational drugs through different routes, such as the sale of personal supplies or theft from pharmacies. Unscrupulous physicians and pharmacists sometimes sell narcotics, barbiturates, similar addictive drugs for recreational use or to maintain a patient's or a customer's addiction. People can become addicted to these drugs even when taking them as part of supervised treatment. Some patients even learn to work the system to their advantage, feeding their addiction by following a complicated route of doctors and drugstores that they piece together.

The Do-It-Yourself Pharmacist

In the movie *My Big Fat Greek Wedding*, Toula Portokalos, the character played by actress Nia Vardalos, tells about how her father used Windex to treat wounds and skin problems such as scrapes, bruises, and warts. Relying on glass cleaner for first aid seems ridiculous to her, until her fiancé uses it to clear up a pimple on his face that appears the day before their wedding.

Like most humor, this tale plays off a core of truth. A lot of people diagnose and treat their own illnesses, often coming up with remedies that are as bizarre as any practiced by physicians in medieval times. Some of these folks seem to have the opinion that no one, not even a physician, knows their bodies better than they do, and that they already have had enough experience with illness to know how to treat themselves. They do not want to spend time and money seeking help from an expert who will only tell them what they already know. Also, many people have a deep-down fear that if they go to the doctor, their illness will turn out to be worse than it would have been if they treated it themselves.

Of course, people have many more health care options these days, and a lot more knowledge about health and hygiene than they would have had in the past. Aside from using OTC medications, people have been able to avoid getting sick simply by knowing how and when diseases take hold in the body. But the added control over their health comes with the ability to damage their health, or at least to waste their time and money, by relying on dangerous or useless self-treatments. The success of the patent medicine industry shows how dangerous it can be to serve as one's own pharmacist.

The type of self-treatment described here goes beyond simply taking an allergy tablet to fight off a case of hay fever. It is closer to the decision to stop taking antibiotics in order to "save some for later." At best, the treatment someone chooses for himself or herself either will succeed or will have no effect, leaving the body free to heal itself. At worst, the treatment will help a disease thrive or weaken the immune system to the point where it cannot fight against an infection.

Nor is the neighborhood drugstore, pharmacy, or grocery the only place people can go to get drugs. For decades, Americans living near the border between the United States and Mexico have traveled south to the pharmacies of Tijuana, Mexicali, Nogales, Nuevo Laredo, and other Mexican border cities. Food and drug laws in Mexico are less stringent about some medicines than are the laws of the United States, and pharmacies can sell many drugs, such as antibiotics, without a written prescription. As attractive as this feature of international commerce is, people from the United States also are drawn to the prices at the Mexican pharmacies, which can be as little as half the cost for the same drugs north of the border. Adding in the cost of a visit to a doctor's office to get the prescription means that people could save a significant amount of money, even with the travel expenses. Both nations have limited the amount of medicine that visitors can take over the border. However, the number of visitors seeking lower-priced, hassle-free drugs still forms a multimillion-dollar-a-year business.

More recently, the Internet has provided a digital bazaar that includes a large number of online pharmacies promising huge discounts on prescription medications. Theoretically, pharmacies are only allowed to accept written prescriptions or phone prescriptions from licensed physicians, preferably ones who practice in the same state. In reality, though, many online pharmacies have worked around these regulations by keeping physicians on their payrolls to review patient orders and, if needed, consult with patients over the phone.

State and federal governments have been slow to craft new regulations for online pharmacies, partly because they do not want to interfere with legitimate trade. Many national pharmacy chains maintain customer sites on the World Wide Web and toll-free phone order lines for prescription refills. And many other pharmacies, some operated by nonprofit organizations such as AARP (the American Association for Retired Persons), provide mail-order discount prescription services. The trick is to curtail the abuse of loopholes in pharmacy law without disrupting this legitimate business.

Dangerous Dosages

The crisis hit the western suburbs of Chicago, Illinois, in October 1982. Seven people, including a 12-year-old girl in Elk Grove Village and three people in the same Arlington Heights family, died a little while after taking the same brand of the pain-and-fever medicine. At first, no one knew that the seven people had taken the drug. But two off-duty firefighters who were listening to their police-and-fire radios heard the name of the drug mentioned while paramedics were relating the victim's symptoms to nearby hospitals. They reported this discovery to their supervisor, who passed it along to the medical and police authorities who were investigating the deaths.

As it turned out, the drug in question was not to blame for the deaths—at least, not directly. The drug was Extra-Strength Tylenol, the brand name of an analgesic called acetaminophen that had been on the market for decades. Its manufacturer, the pharmaceutical giant Johnson & Johnson, promoted the drug as a safe and effective alternative to aspirin, and it had developed the extra-strength version of the drug to appeal to customers who did not want to take two capsules at a time. Since all the victims had died after taking the painkiller, investigators tested the remaining capsules. Each capsule contained 65 milligrams of cyanide, a poison. Since it only takes about seven micrograms, or seven-millionths of a gram, of cyanide to kill an adult, each capsule contained enough poison to kill more than 10,000 people.

Further investigation only deepened the mystery. The bottle of tainted Tylenol had come from four different lots of the painkiller, but only a few bottles from each lot contained the deadly capsules. In addition, the number of tainted pills in each of these bottles ranged from just a few to as many as 10. And while the first assumption was that Johnson & Johnson's two Tylenol manufacturing plants could have accidentally mixed the poison in with the drug, there actually was no way that the cyanide could have been added in the factories. McNeil Consumer Products, the Johnson & Johnson subsidiary company that made Tylenol, did not make any products that contained cyanide, and none of its suppliers could have accidentally included the poison in the raw materials they sold. The only explanation for the huge amount of poison in the pills was sabotage.

The most likely explanation was that somebody bought bottles of Extra-Strength Tylenol at random in different drugstores, added the cyanide, and placed the altered drugs on shelves in stores where they would most likely be bought quickly. No one knows who was responsible for poisoning the drugs, though a man who was arrested and sentenced to prison for 20 years after he attempted to extort $1 million from McNeil was one of the strongest suspects in the case. What is certain is that the poisoner had an easy time adding the cyanide. The closest thing to tamper-resistant packaging in those days was a child safety cap that federal law required on prescription and OTC medications. Otherwise, the only thing that separated the customer from a product was a box flap that may have been glued shut or, possibly, a foil "freshness seal" on a bottle. Since the drug was a powder contained in a shell much like a plastic Easter egg, the poisoner would have been able to open the capsule, mix in the cyanide, and reassemble the capsule with little effort. Once he or she finished this task and returned the pills to their packaging, no one would have been able to detect the tampering.

When the cause of the poisoning became known, Johnson & Johnson pulled the entire supply of Tylenol off the market, spending more than $100 million to recall the drug. They also began developing new methods for making and packaging their product, a lead that other companies followed, as well as food and beverage makers. From blister packs of throat lozenges to pop-up buttons on the lids of salsa bottles, the use of most tamper-resistant or tamper-evident packaging got started as a result of the of terror the poisoning created.

Prescription-Drug Addiction

It seems to be a disease of the rich and famous: Every year, some well-known celebrities or sports figures will check into a drug rehab center to beat addiction to painkillers. Others will be arrested with prescription narcotics in their possession that they bought illegally. Usually, their addiction will be the result of a bad accident or a painful operation for which they first received the drugs. The problems start when they find themselves unable or unwilling to go through the effects of coming off the drugs.

Prescription-drug addiction is a serious problem for many patients. Chemically, there is nothing inherently "bad" about illegal drugs, just as there is nothing inherently "good" about prescription and OTC drugs. The problems come from how these chemical compounds react with the mind and body of the people who take them. Many illegal drugs, in fact, started out as pharmaceuticals. Remember, the scientist who discovered heroin considered it a safe, nonaddictive alternative painkiller to morphine, until he became addicted to it. The hallucinogen *phencyclidine* (PCP) was created in the 1950s and used for decades as a horse tranquilizer. It got the nickname *angel dust* because of the extreme sense of euphoria it creates in humans—an effect probably discovered by accident—but it became notorious for the extreme bursts of violence it also creates in many of the people who take it.

Unfortunately, many valuable prescription drugs also carry a high risk of addiction. Physicians have to get a special permit from the Food and Drug Administration to prescribe any of these narcotic drugs, and they—as well as the pharmacists who supply the drugs—have to submit paperwork tracking each of these prescriptions. This paper trail is why patients who get prescriptions filled for painkillers such as Vicodin (a brand-name version of hydrocodone) must sign for their drugs.

One way people have managed to get around the restrictions on prescribing narcotics has been to go to more than one physician and one pharmacy. Because of the tight tracking requirements, these people will use false names with each new doctor and each pharmacy. In itself, this practice is illegal, whether or not the patient is trying to get narcotic or nonnarcotic drugs. Another way is to find a physician or a pharmacist who is willing to prescribe these painkillers and falsify records to show that these patients needed the drugs. Of course, a more direct way to get the drugs is either to steal them or to buy them from people who have their own prescriptions. All of the methods are equally illegal, but, unfortunately, they also are equally effective.

Just as the drugs do not have to be painkillers, people do not have to deliberately seek to get high in order to become addicted. Many patients, especially older people, go from one physician to another to treat legitimate maladies. They may go to one physician to treat one group of illnesses and to another to treat a different group. They may lose their temper with one physician and go to another without having their medical records sent along. Some patients may even think that they will end up becoming healthier by combining more than one treatment method. Like people who seek painkillers illegally, these patients will get multiple prescriptions for the same or similar drugs and fill them at separate pharmacies.

The problem with this overreliance on medicine comes when people overdose on a medication, either through taking too much of one drug or through taking two drugs that interact and enhance each other's side effects (as mentioned in Chapter 12). There are countless ways in which people can harm themselves by mixing medications this way. The consequences include heart or nerve damage, breathing problems, hallucinations, and a host of other physical and psychological injuries. With luck, people can overcome these effects by getting off the medicines that caused the interactions, possibly with the assistance of other drugs that can help repair the damage. The true risk, though, is that these results will be permanent, leading to further reliance on medications simply to stay alive.

18

DISTRIBUTION WOES

Medicines cannot do the work they are designed to do unless they get from the factory to the marketplace. Despite their critical role in restoring and maintaining the health of those who take them, though, medicines are a commodity, and they are subject to the same rules of commerce that affect any other commodity. A company that develops a highly profitable drug will be reluctant to bring that drug to market, regardless of the number of lives it could save, if the disease it treats affects only a small group of people. Likewise, a drug that costs a lot of time and effort to make will not earn a large profit for its man-ufacturers, even if millions of people demand it.

For pharmaceutical companies, an ideal drug is one like Viagra, a treatment for male sexual impotency that Pfizer, Inc., began sell-ing in the 1990s. Viagra sold for $10 a pill when it first hit the mar-ket and found a ready customer base: millions of older men who had developed a common condition called erectile dysfunction, in which the blood vessels of the penis cannot remain dilated long enough to sustain an erection. Within weeks, Viagra became the best-selling new drug in history, eventually earning billions of dollars for Pfizer. But such blockbuster drugs are rare, and most companies have to be contented with the smaller but steady profits of standard medicines such as antibiotics, antidepressants, and other, more commonly used pharmaceuticals.

On the opposite end of the pharmaceutical spectrum are vaccines for common diseases, such as influenza, rabies, and the eight "child-hood diseases": chickenpox, the vaccine for which came out in the mid-

1990s; diphtheria, a respiratory infection that creates huge amounts of deadly toxins in the body; measles; mumps; pertussis, or whooping cough; pneumococcal disease, which causes potentially fatal forms of pneumonia and meningitis; rubella, also known as German measles; and tetanus. Although these diseases are common enough to create a permanent demand for their vaccines, drug companies do not earn great amounts of money from supplying these shots. While most vaccines have long passed the point where they are covered by patents, the costs of making the vaccines are high enough, and the pressure to keep prices low is great enough, to discourage all but a few companies from making these drugs on a regular basis. Combined with the tight regulations placed on these companies, this fact of business life can lead to a lot of trouble.

The Flu Vaccine Shortage of Y2K

The flu vaccine proved to be one of the great success stories of the 20th century. Its creation dramatically reduced the number of people who came down with influenza every year, saving the lives of those who might not have survived the disease and saving the world's economy billions of dollars every year that might have been lost when sick workers stayed home. As long as people were not allergic to eggs—which served as the generators for the weakened flu virus—they could count on receiving their yearly shot against the flu—unless the flu shot was not available. That happened in the United States during the final year of the 20th century, when the system for making flu vaccines almost broke down. By the 1990s, only four pharmaceutical companies made vaccines, and one of those companies stopped making the shots shortly before the end of the decade. Flu vaccines are not a big moneymaker: The highest price anyone pays for the shot is $30 in a physician's office, and a huge number of people get vaccinated at low-cost flu-shot clinics where they can pay as little as eight dollars. Also, making flu vaccines involves following procedures set out by the Food and Drug Administration.

Still, the three remaining manufacturers seemed to be able to keep producing the 75 million doses of the vaccine that the United States required in 1999. That figure may not seem like enough—it represents just a little more than one-quarter of the population—but it is enough to cover the people who are most likely to come down with the flu every year, including the people who are most likely to die from the disease.

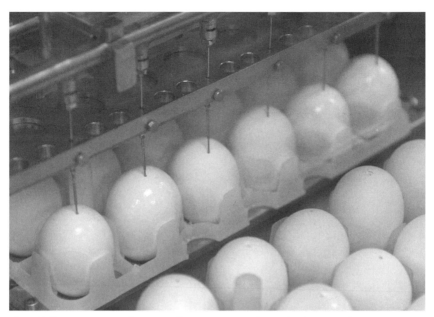

Though flu vaccine suppliers usually can meet each year's demand, there was a serious shortage in the year 2000. [Aventis Pasteur]

The situation suddenly became worse in 2000, when FDA inspectors found that one of the three vaccine makers was not "in compliance" with the agency's rules for making the vaccine. Neither the FDA nor the drug company publicly said how the firm had fallen out of compliance with the regulations, but the company had to shut down its factory for more than a year in order to improve conditions. The other two companies increased their production to exploit this sudden opportunity, but they could not hope to fill the gap. With half of its flu vaccine producers out of the market, the United States found itself with only two-thirds the number of shots—50 million doses—that it needed. Worse, the two remaining vaccine manufacturers could not deliver these shots all at once. The best they could do was send out batches throughout the course of flu-shot season, which runs from roughly mid-September to mid-February, a period from a little before to halfway through the time that influenza usually hits the nation.

Because of the vaccine shortage, the FDA asked the public to start a voluntary self-rationing program early in the 2000–01 flu season. Adults between 18 and 45 are at lowest risk of dying or suffering long-term harm from the flu, so they were asked to hold off on getting a shot. The most critical task was to immunize infants, young children, and the elderly, all of whose immune systems were most likely to succumb to the virus. Fortunately, the strains of flu that hit during the 2000–01 season were not particularly deadly, and the third vaccine manufacturer was able to return its factory to production in time to prevent another shortage during the following season.

Though the flu vaccine shortage highlighted the nation's vulnerability to large-scale epidemics, the news was not a surprise to its public-health officials. Vaccine shortages of all types have been a problem both for the United States and for the rest of the world for decades.

Recent examples of these shortages include a prolonged period in which U.S. state health authorities had to deal with partial droughts of vaccines that covered the eight childhood illnesses. Because these eight diseases are some of the most common, the most deadly, and the most easily transmitted childhood illnesses, school districts throughout the nation require students to be immunized against them before or soon after starting school. But, as with the influenza vaccine, only a handful of companies made these drugs—in fact, only one company, Merck and Co., Inc., made the chicken pox vaccine, which it began producing in 1995.

The shortages caused some dramatic shifts in the way the states handled childhood immunization. Many states reported deliveries only every few months. In 2002 health agencies in 49 of the 50 states said they were forced to ration these vaccines, sending the greatest amount to the cities and counties where they were likely to do the most good. As a result, many children simply had to go without their vaccinations, and school districts had to alter their immunization requirements to compensate. Fortunately, the shortage did not seem to lead to an immediate outbreak of these diseases, but health officials throughout the nation said students who did not receive their shots would be at great risk in case of a future epidemic.

Supply and Demand

In a way, shortages such as these are the result of humanity's success in inoculating itself against disease. All the microbes for which there are vaccinations—the ones that cause flu, rabies, polio, smallpox, tetanus, and the rest—once were some of the most deadly threats that people faced in their lives. The average life expectancy of a boy or girl born in the United States just before 1900 was about 45 years. This figure did not mean that most people died when they were 45. Plenty of people lived long lives, and others did not die until they were in their late 50s or 60s. However, disease claimed many children before they had a chance to reach adulthood, and many adults succumbed to epidemics for which there were no cures or reliable vaccines until much later.

Some of these diseases are ones that people in nations with advanced health care systems no longer worry about. For example, yellow fever, a viral disease that attacks the liver, once killed hundreds of thousands of people around the world every decade, including in the Americas from Canada to South America. Though the virus that caused the disease was native to equatorial Africa, a species of mosquito called *Aedes aegypti* carried it around the world in the holds of sailing ships. Anywhere the mosquito could breed, people were at risk of contracting the disease. The discovery of a vaccine against the disease, combined with insect-control efforts, either eliminated yellow fever or brought it under control in most urban areas throughout the world, and in rural areas in developed nations such as the United States and Canada. As with most diseases, yellow fever still exists, but it no longer poses quite the same threat.

In a way, though, successes such as this were unfortunate. Public health workers and officials often say that getting close to wiping out a disease, but not quite getting it all, may be worse than allowing the disease to progress normally. Whenever people think that medical science has conquered a disease, they tend to cut back on the measures that conquered it. Why spend money, they think, preventing something that does not seem to be a threat anymore? At the same time, when drug companies see a drop in sales of a vaccine, they naturally tend to slow down or stop producing it. After all, it does no one any good for the companies to make vaccines that will only sit in warehouses or on storage shelves. Not only will the companies not make money on these unsold vaccines, but the drugs likely will lose their potency before anyone needs to use them. Vaccines have a limited shelf life, and even the longest-lasting eventually will lose the ability to trigger the immune system.

Other shortages come not from a lack of production but from difficulties in distribution. Healthy supplies of a vaccine do not do anyone any good if there is no way to get them to the people who need them. This fact of life is felt especially hard in underdeveloped nations of South America, Africa, and Asia, particularly in nations going through periods of civil war, drought, or other calamities. Many of these nations simply cannot afford to make or bring in the medicines they need. Others have governments that are so chaotic or corrupt that there is no guarantee any drug shipments will arrive at their intended destinations. International groups, such as the United Nations and nonprofit religious and humanitarian organizations, as well as national governments, have programs to bring medicines and other forms of aid to these nations, as well as physicians to treat the sick and work with doctors in these nations.

Production Problems

Shortages are not a problem for every type of drug, of course. There has never been a shortage of aspirin, nor has anyone suffered from a lack of penicillin or other antibiotics since the late 1940s. Drugs such as these are both cheap to produce and in high demand by customers, making them products that drug companies are happy to produce. And even when drugs are expensive to produce or have little demand, there would not be any risk of shortages if a few drug companies were willing to maintain the necessary production lines on a standby basis, ready to start work once the need for those drugs arose. Right?

Well, not exactly. The fact is, by the time people realize that they need a rarely used drug, they barely have enough time to stop an outbreak or treat a condition—provided the drug is available. If a company has to start up a production line and produce the drug from scratch, it may not be able to get the drug to its intended patients in time. Consider the production schedule for making each year's flu vaccine, which Chapter 10 covers. From the time the U.S. Centers for Disease Control and Prevention determines which strains of influenza most likely will strike the nation, the three companies that make the vaccine take nearly two-thirds of a year to prepare the shots for shipment. The production time for other vaccines is even longer, in some cases lasting longer than a year. Many diseases could run their course in their original hosts and infect countless others before their vaccines were ready.

There would be other problems with trying to maintain such a "just in case we need it" production line. First, of course, would be the cost of setting up such a facility. A drug factory is a multimillion-dollar installation, with acres of floor space, miles of plumbing, and some of the most expensive computer-control equipment in the world. They also have to be highly secure facilities, given the large amounts of potentially hazardous chemicals that pass in and out through their doors. Even the finished products have to be treated with a high level of security, if only to prevent the theft of the more expensive pharmaceuticals.

Assume for a moment, though, that a pharmaceutical company was willing to set up a production facility for a couple of these rarely used drugs. The cost of this facility would not stop piling up once construction was finished. The company would have to hire employees and security guards to maintain and protect the facility while it was sitting idle, pay its property taxes and utility fees, and every now and then inspect it to make sure it would be ready to go into service when needed. If the time came when the facility was needed, the company first would have to make sure the equipment was ready to go (and fix any machinery that was not working), hire or transfer people to get it running, order the ingredients for the drug, and prove to the FDA that the facility was ready to go into production. All this activity would add to the time it took to ship the first batch of medicine, and any problems before or during the production period would add to the delay.

In reality, this type of operation is impractical. No company can afford to build factories that spend most of their time sitting idle, just as no company really can afford to make drugs that have little or no profit potential. There are exceptions to this rule, of course: the orphan drugs that treat diseases that affect a relatively low number of people (defined as 200,000 people or fewer in the United States). But the tax breaks, the development grants, and the seven-year exclusive-use clause granted by the nation's Orphan Drug Act provide only so much encouragement for drug companies to create and produce these drugs. Sooner or later, economics will force them to decide whether or not to keep a drug going.

When the vaccine shortages of the late 20th and early 21st centuries pointed out the United States's vulnerability, officials from the Institute of Medicine (a research group supported by the National Academy of Sciences) proposed a solution to cover this gap. In a 1993 report the institute suggested establishing a national vaccine authority both to manufacture vaccines in a government-run facility and to sponsor research into new vaccines and new vaccination methods. The Institute focused on the need for a vaccine authority because, among other reasons, the Orphan Drug Act does not cover vaccines, nor was there any legislation to establish a similar program for vaccines. But the national vaccine authority idea went nowhere until after the terrorist attacks of September 11, 2001, and the subsequent "anthrax letter" scare. With new attention being given to the possibility of bioterrorism attacks, the institute's president, Kenneth Shine, began promoting the idea of a government-run vaccine program more forcefully.

Naturally, pharmaceutical companies have opposed such a government agency. Not only do they not want to have the federal government as a competitor, but also they say they will be able to meet the need for vaccines once the nation sorts out its health care priorities. In 2002, drug firms and the pharmaceutical industry's lobbying group said the nation's vaccine shortages were partly the result of complacency—

from the centuries of success in treating and eradicating disease—and partly the result of some federal vaccine-purchase programs that forced prices so low that producers were discouraged from making the drugs. The programs, one industry official said, effectively created caps on the prices the companies could charge for their vaccines.

There also is a philosophical issue that has to be considered: Is establishing a new government agency truly the best solution for such a health care problem as the vaccine shortage? Many people in and outside of the government would argue that the problem is too big for anyone but the government to handle. Not only would the government have the resources to solve the problem—in the form of taxpayers' money and government research expertise—but it would be in a position. to produce vaccines, stockpile them, maintain them, and distribute them as rapidly as possible. However, just as many people would say that a new government bureaucracy would be the least effective means of handling the problem. Private pharmaceutical companies, they would argue, already are set up to make the vaccines the world needs, and they already have efficient distribution methods in place.

Regardless of which solution may win out—that is, if either one ever does—it is clear that the process of producing vaccines, as well as many other drugs, will have to be improved. If not, a shortage may strike just when the drugs are needed most.

19

FUTURE TRENDS IN PHARMACOLOGY

Modern medicines can be dangerous. They can sicken or kill people who are allergic to them. They can help make dangerous microbes stronger if people misuse them, and they can trigger years of addiction if people abuse them. Yet, when people use them properly, most pharmaceutical drugs are safe and effective, more so than almost any other medicine ever used. The only exceptions might be the traditional, plant-based medicines that people have used for thousands of years, which drug researchers are examining as potential sources of future drugs.

The vast improvement in medicine—which has helped increase the average lifespan of people throughout the world—came from more than two centuries of scientific research into disease, the immune system, and the chemical nature of drugs. As has happened in all other fields of science, this research revealed new areas to be explored and developed. In the last decades of the 20th century, scientists began working on forms of health care that seemed to have come from science fiction rather than science. Turning bacteria into insulin factories was one of the results of this work. There have been many others.

For instance, the Human Genome Project of the 1990s was the most ambitious scientific quest in history. A *genome* is the entire list of genes that are present in the DNA of a particular species, along with their location on that species' chromosomes. Determining this information, a process called *sequencing*, gives scientists an idea of which genes are responsible for hereditary traits, such as eye color, and hereditary malfunctions, such as some types of birth defect or common maladies such as nearsightedness. Although scientists working in separate nations had studied the structure of human, animal, and plant genes for decades, in 1990 a group of nations joined to form the Human Genome Organization, which coordinated this work and helped scientists share their discoveries with each other.

The goal seemed overwhelming; many people thought the project would take at least 15 years to accomplish. Even though DNA contains only four bases—adenine, cytosine, guanine, and thymine—each organism's genetic code mixes these bases in tens of thousands of combinations. When they started, the scientists who worked on the human genome estimated they would have to identify and map more than 3 billion bases within 50,000 to 100,000 genes. The first preliminary map of the genome came out three years later, when a team of French scientists released a rough version of the genome showing a relative handful of genes that they had identified and located. By the late 1990s scientists had identified only 7,000 genes and had figured out the locations of only 5,000 of these.

Then, at the turn of the millennium, an independent company called Celera Genomics announced that it had finished the task of sequencing the human genome using advanced analysis equipment and a highly powerful supercomputer. Naturally, scientists with the Human Genome Project checked the Celera Genomics data, but they ended up agreeing that the small research company had succeeded in completing the task about five years earlier than had been expected. The result was that a little more than 32,000 genes determined the physical characteristics of human beings; there were more strings of bases on DNA than were in these genes, but these were little more than "junk code" that had accumulated during millions of years of evolution. (Later, other scientists suggested that much of what appeared to be "junk code" actually might form genes that the genome researchers had not recognized.)

Clues from the Genome

But so what? What drove these scientists to figure out how much of our DNA shapes what we are and where these genes are?

The point of the decade-long research project was to gain a better understanding of how the body works and to figure out ways for doctors to craft treatments and medications to their patients the way a tailor can fit a suit of clothes to a particular customer. Knowing ahead of time that patients cannot tolerate certain drugs or how their immune system responds to a type of microbe could help speed up recovery times or prevent illnesses from developing in the first place. It might even be possible one day to correct some genetic abnormalities before a child is born.

The knowledge of human and animal genetics was yielding many benefits before the Human Genome Project got under way. Humans and other mammals share similar biological makeups, but there are many differences. A drug might work in a culture dish and in an experimental animal, but then fail in a human being. These differences can be extreme: There are drugs that will cure all types of cancer in mice without producing the same effect on human tumors. But what if human genes could be grafted into mice or other laboratory animals? Drug researchers might be able to find out how human cells react to new drugs without having to wait until the start of human clinical tests. As late as the middle of the 1980s, such an idea was restricted to the pages and films of science fiction. These days, though, such *transgenic animals* are common throughout the field of medical research.

Transgenic animals carry fragments of the DNA of other species within their cells. These fragments, called *transgenes,* can come from any animal species and are placed within the fertilized egg cell of another species using microscopic needles. The new genetic material works its way into the egg cell's DNA; as the egg divides and develops into a complete organism, the transgene will influence how some of its cells or organs develop. The method is similar to the recombinant DNA technique for turning bacteria into insulin-producing factories.

Scientists have used transgenic mice to study diseases that could only be seen in larger animals before the 1990s. For example, normal mice do not develop a disease called hepatitis B, but chimpanzees do. Chimpanzees are far more expensive and difficult to care for than mice are, though, and it takes them longer to show symptoms of the disease and to respond to treatment. With the development of transgenic mice, scientists have been able to conduct more research into the disease, since they can substitute the mice for the apes. Other genetic engineering projects have produced mice that are more sensitive than normal to *carcinogens,* chemicals and other substances in the environment that can cause cancer. Since it is easier to detect the presence of carcinogens in an area by testing samples on these highly sensitive mice, researchers can now use fewer animals to identify cancer hazards, but it is easier to study the progression of cancer and determine if potential cancer drugs will succeed or fail.

Transgenic animals also have given researchers the opportunity to study diseases that once were hard to analyze. Alzheimer's disease is one of the most terrifying maladies that can strike a person. It is a brain disorder that causes a steadily increasing loss of memory and an accompanying loss of other brain functions. It also is a disease that affects more than just its victims: The family and friends of Alzheimer's patients find themselves having to cope with the fact that a person they have known and loved for years no longer can remember them. Research into the disease was slow and expensive because scientists could only study it in older primates, such as chimpanzees, as these animals were the only ones who developed the disease the way human beings did. There was no similar disorder in rodents—until scientists developed a strain of transgenic mice that could develop Alzheimer's. Once that strain arrived, scientists were able to study the disease in whole generations of mice in a matter of months, rather than years, as was necessary in chimps.

No one knows just how much of a difference the ability to read the genome and manipulate genetic codes will make to biomedical research. Medical experts say that such abilities are certain to bring major changes in the study of aging, birth defects, cancer, allergies, autoimmune diseases, infectious diseases, and environmental health. Indeed, through the final years of the 20th century, such knowledge helped researchers learn many new things about how diseases develop and how to cure them. However, it also posed a number of scientific and ethical dilemmas that people still have to solve.

One of the most serious of these dilemmas is the issue of *stem cell* research. Stem cells are primitive, *undifferentiated* cells that develop into the specialized cells that form bones, blood, hair, and internal organs. All creatures start out as a mass of stem cells created after a sperm cell and an egg join to form a complete *zygote*, which divides and grows into a complete organism during *gestation*. Masses of stem cells that are in the process of sorting themselves into different types of body tissue are called *embryos;* after the cells have more or less settled down into their final forms, the developing infant is called a *fetus.* In humans, the transition from embryo to fetus takes place around the end of the second month of pregnancy, after which there are dramatically fewer stem cells. By the end of pregnancy, about the only stem cells left in the body are those in the bone marrow that develop into *erythrocytes* (red blood cells).

Because stem cells can turn into any other form of body cell, many medical researchers have experimented with turning them into therapeutic drugs that could cure maladies ranging from Parkinson's disease, a

HUMAN GENOME

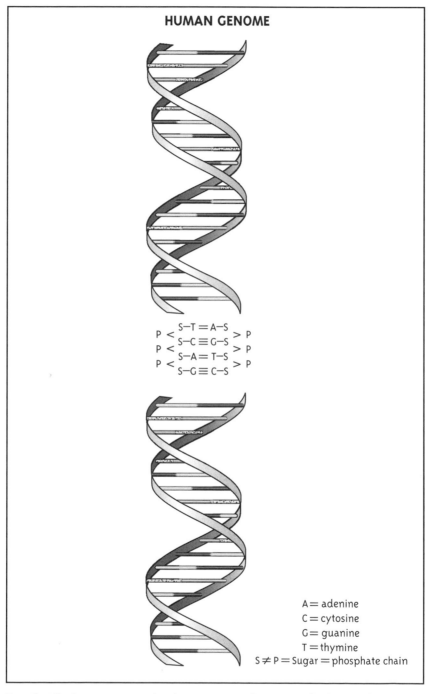

$$P < {S-T = A-S \atop S-C \equiv G-S} > P$$
$$P < {S-A = T-S \atop S-G \equiv C-S} > P$$

A = adenine
C = cytosine
G = guanine
T = thymine
S ≠ P = Sugar = phosphate chain

Now that the human genome has been sequenced, many medical researchers believe they have the genetic road map they need to find treatments for hereditary illnesses and other maladies.

breakdown in the brain's motor control centers, to diabetes. Physicians already use transplants of human stem cells, the ones in the bone marrow that turn into erythrocytes, to replace blood cells lost in patients who develop some forms of cancer. However, these types of stem cells already are programmed to turn into erythrocytes. Other therapeutic uses would require human stem cells that were even simpler in construction, but the only way to get such cells would be to harvest them from undeveloped embryos or from fetuses in their earliest stages of development.

Many people find appalling the thought of harvesting embryos or fetuses for their stem cells. In most cases these cells would come from embryos and fetuses following an abortion, which many people already object to on religious or philosophical grounds. These people believe that allowing scientists to extract stem cells for use in research and as medicine would turn what they see as an already repugnant act into something even worse: a devaluation of human life into a source of "spare parts." There are similar objections to another method for generating stem cells—fertilizing donated eggs and sperm in a laboratory, then stopping the development of the embryo before the stem cells begin to specialize. Many people believe that life begins at conception, whether conception takes place in a woman's body or in a test tube.

Many other people, though, believe that the issue of when life begins depends on the development of the fetus and its ability to live outside its mother's womb. Their opinion is that the fetus is not truly an individual until it reaches a certain stage of physical development and brain activity. Therefore, people who hold this view believe there is no reason not to use these stem cells, especially since doing so will heal and prolong the lives of so many people.

The debate over the stem cell issue has been almost as strident, at times, as the debate over abortion. Some scientists have attempted to cancel out both sides' arguments by perfecting other ways of getting stem cells, such as by extracting them from the umbilical cords of newborns. However, the issue promises to generate controversy for years to come.

Old Enemies Become Unlikely Allies

Scientists used computers to design many of the new drugs that emerged during the 1990s and early 2000s. Once drug researchers know the molecular structure of the microbe they want to attack, they can use a computer to create and analyze compounds that can fit into that structure and either break it apart or shut it down. That is, most of the time, after a long, tedious, and complicated process of designing structures they think will work and then redesigning them when these molecules turn out not to function as they should have.

Nature, however, has been working on just this problem for millions of years, and it long ago developed a set of tools for attacking microbes: other microbes. Not only have microbes learned how to exploit weaknesses in humans, animals, and plants, but they also have developed ways to keep other microbes from doing the same thing. Remember, before penicillin became a drug it was part of the antibacterial arsenal of the *penicillium* fungus. Just as bacteria-killing poisons like this became some of the world's most powerful pharmaceuticals, scientists have been searching for ways to turn the natural warfare between microbes to humanity's benefit.

One focus of this type of research is a group of viruses called *bacteriophages*. Though the name means "bacteria eater," bacteriophages actually have the same goal as any other virus: to penetrate a cell and reprogram it to make more viruses. The problem with bacteria is that, like plant cells, they have very tough cellular walls, far tougher than the walls of animal cells. Bacteriophages, though, developed a structure shaped something like a syringe to puncture the cell wall and inject the virus's genetic code. Researchers think that it might be possible one day to engineer viruses that attack specific bacteria—drug-resistant *Staphylococcus* or *Streptococcus*, for example—without harming human beings or infecting other, possibly beneficial microbes.

Actually, bacteriophage research dates back to the end of the 19th century, when medical researchers recognized that something was capable of killing whole colonies of bacteria. Over the next 40 years, scientists tested various methods of bacteriophage therapy with different levels of success. The dawn of the antibiotic era put a temporary end to most of this research that lasted until the problem of antibiotic resistance forced scientists to look elsewhere for new drugs. Researchers know so much more about viruses these days that bacteriophage therapy has a better chance of succeeding than it did in the past. It may not even be necessary to engineer an entire group of viruses in order to benefit from their attack methods. A group of researchers at Texas A&M University discovered that one group of bacteriophages produced a protein that prevents bacteria from forming and repairing cell walls as they grow. If this protein could be produced in large enough quantities, the scientists said, it could form the basis of a new group of antibiotics.

Who Will Make Our Drugs?

Even if our new knowledge about the genome leads to tailored medicines and new forms of therapy, even if scientists can turn germs into pharmaceuticals, there will never be an end to the need for new drugs or the desire to learn more about the many threats to health that people have to deal with. What will be interesting to see in the years ahead is exactly where our new drugs will come from. When drugs came from plant, mineral, and animal sources, drug companies often maintained their own farms and quarries to ensure a steady supply. When fungi and bacteria began providing drugs, pharmaceutical companies devoted whole laboratories to growing and preserving the proper strains of these microbes.

Future drug sources may require drug firms to enter entirely new lines of work. Most fish, for instance, excrete a coat of slime beneath their outer skin as insulation and to help keep themselves clean. But the Arabian saltwater catfish secretes a gel-like substance that helps it to heal wounds quickly by sealing and protecting them from dirty water. When biologists analyzed the catfish's slime, they discovered it contains 60 different proteins that speed up the healing process. Naturally, some drug companies began working with catfish slime to see if they could turn it into a drug that helps mend sores and wounds in people who do not heal well—burn victims, diabetics, the elderly, and AIDS patients. The trick would be to produce the same type of proteins in the same general concentration as those found in the catfish slime. If this feat could not be accomplished in a lab, the drug company that succeeded might have to start its own Arabian saltwater catfish farm.

More important, though, is the matter of who will provide these drugs. There are fewer large drug companies today than there were at the start of the 1990s, not because many firms went out of business, but because many firms merged to create giant corporations with widely diversified product lines and the ability to do more research than any of the individual companies could have performed. At the same time, many small drug companies began to supply the new market for genetically engineered pharmaceuticals. By focusing on just a few types of drugs, these firms have been able to attain a level of success once reserved for the world's largest manufacturers. Whether the large firms, the small firms, or a combination of both ends up supplying the world's pharmaceutical supplies remains to be seen.

But who is to say that the future of modern medicines depends solely on drug companies? If the scientists who helped decode the

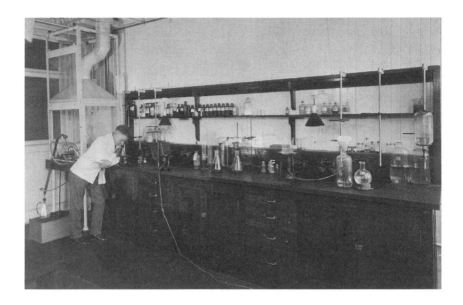

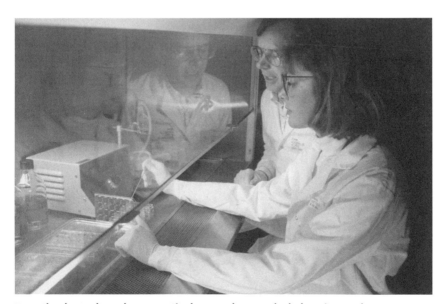

From the days when pharmaceutical researchers worked alone in wooden laboratories to modern times, when large teams have access to high-tech equipment, drug companies have invested enormous amounts of time and money in developing new medicines. [Courtesy Eli Lilly and Company]

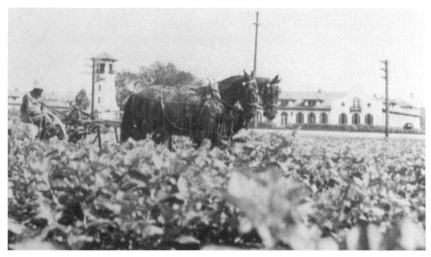

During World War I Eli Lilly raised its own belladonna crops, including this one in Greenfield, Indiana. Such extreme measures of keeping the flow of raw materials coming in are rare, and companies these days get nearly all of their ingredients from independent suppliers. [Courtesy Eli Lilly and Company]

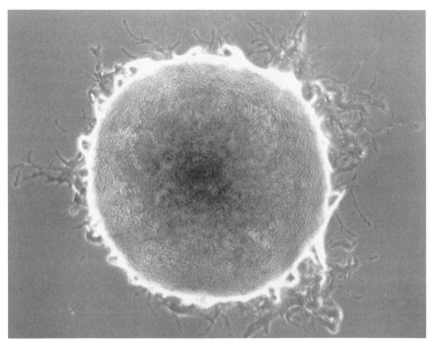

Microbes, such as this *Lysobacter* soil bacterium, are likely to be sources of new drugs in years to come. [Brad Borlee, Department of Plant Pathology, University of Wisconsin—Madison]

human genome are right, the day may come when each patient receives drugs tailor-made for his or her physiology. If that day arrives, the person most responsible for compounding modern medicines might well be someone like the old-time neighborhood pharmacist, a skilled professional who mixes the proper pills and potions in a well-equipped laboratory behind the pharmacy counter.

GLOSSARY

acetylcholine   One of the body's neurotransmitters.

acetylsalicylic acid   *See* ASPIRIN.

acquired immunodeficiency syndrome (AIDS)   A life-threatening disease that attacks the human body's immune system. AIDS is the final stage of an infection by the human immunodeficiency virus.

addiction   In medicine, a physical or psychological dependency on a chemical substance.

adenosine   One of the three chemical bases present in DNA and RNA.

Aedes aegypti   A species of mosquito that carries the yellow fever virus.

agar   A form of red seaweed jelly that researchers use to grow bacteria.

AIDS   *See* ACQUIRED IMMUNODEFICIENCY SYNDROME.

alimentary canal   The tube running from the lips to the rectum through which people and animals take in food, digest it, and eliminate solid waste.

allergen   Any material that causes or reveals an allergy in a person or an animal.

allergy   An unusual response of the immune system to a normally nonthreatening substance.

amino acid   A chemical compound that serves as a basic building block of protein molecules.

amphetamine   A potentially addictive chemical that increases the body's metabolic rate. It can also relieve nasal congestion or reduce a person's appetite. Amphetamines also are known as "speed."

analgesic   A drug that blocks or dulls pain.

anaphylactic shock   A severe, potentially fatal allergic reaction that causes its victim to lose consciousness. Sometimes, the only treatment for cases of anaphylactic shock is an immediate injection of epinephrine.

anecdotal evidence   Stories from patients or doctors about the success of a particular drug or treatment method that supposedly prove its worth. Because such stories are, at best, influenced by personal opinion—and, at worst, are made up—anecdotal evidence is not considered by regulatory agencies that approve drugs.

anemia   A lower-than-average level of leukocytes in the blood.

anesthesia   The loss of pain or other feeling in the body or in one area of the body.

anesthetic   A chemical or other method that causes anesthesia.

angel dust   *See* PHENCYCLIDINE.

aniline dye   An artificial dye that was used to stain microbes for microscopic examination and later became a vehicle for delivering drugs to microbes.

antacid   A substance that neutralizes acids, especially one that eliminates excess digestive acids in humans.

anthrax   An infectious, potentially fatal disease caused by the anthracis bacteria.

antianxiety   A medicinal drug that counteracts feelings of anxiety or tension.

antibiotic   A chemical compound made by a living organism that kills bacteria or stops their growth.

antibody   A protein produced in the body by white blood cells that recognizes a specific foreign molecule and either destroys or deactivates it.

antidepressant   A drug that combats clinical or other forms of depression.

antigen   Any form of protein that triggers the immune system to produce antibodies.

antihistamine   A drug that treats colds, hay fever, and some allergies by interfering with the action of HISTAMINES.

antipsychotic   A drug that counteracts the chemical causes of psychosis.

antipyretic   A drug that reduces or eliminates fevers. The term *pyretic* stems from *pyr*, the Greek word for fire.

antiseptic   Something that either is able to prevent disease or is not favorable to the growth of disease organisms.

antiseptic surgery   Surgical methods adopted since the middle of the 19th century that prevent the spread of disease in the operating room.

antiviral   A drug or other substance that is able to suppress or kill viruses.

apothecary   An old term for pharmacist.

arsenic   A poisonous metal that has been used as a medicine.

arteriosclerosis   A thickening or hardening of the walls of the arteries that causes a decreased level of blood circulation.

artery   A blood vessel that carries blood away from the heart.

Aspergillis   A fungus that, like *Penicillium*, produces penicillin.

aspirin   An over-the-counter fever reducer and painkiller that is the best-selling drug in the world. Also known as acetylsalicylic acid.

atom   The smallest part of an element that has all the chemical properties of that element. Atoms are the building blocks of all matter.

autoimmune disease   A medical condition in which the body's immune system attacks the body's own cells and organs.

bacteria   Single-celled organisms that are smaller and simpler forms of life than plant and animal cells. The DNA of a bacterium is not organized in a separate, organized nucleus, but in a general area of the bacterium's interior called a nucleoid.

bacteriologist   A scientist who studies bacteria and devises means to combat them.

bacteriophage   A virus that has evolved to attack bacteria.

bacterium   Singular form of the word BACTERIA.

barbiturate   A sedative that can calm people or send them to sleep. Barbiturates are potentially addictive.

base   In genetics, one of the chemicals in DNA and RNA that form genes.

B complex   A group of vitamins that includes biotin, cobalamin (B-12), folic acid, niacin, pyridoxine, pantothenic acid (B-6), riboflavin (B-2), and thiamin (B-1).

bezoar stones   Solid masses of hair and other material that form in the stomachs of animals, particularly in the wild bezoar goats of the Greek islands and the Near East. Bezoar stones were thought to have the power to neutralize poisons.

bile   A fluid produced by the liver that helps digest food and absorb fats.

bile, black   One of the bodily humors that once were thought to regulate the health of the body. Black bile supposedly controlled mood, and an excess of this liquid caused depression.

bile, yellow   Another of the bodily humors that were thought to regulate health. Fevers were considered to be the result of too much yellow bile. Some actual bile pigments are naturally yellow in color.

biochemical   Related to the chemical activity within living organisms.

biochemist   A scientist who specializes in the field of biochemistry.

biochemistry   The study of the chemical processes that take place within living organisms.

bipolar disorder   A form of mental illness in which a person's mood alternates between periods of extreme elation, or mania, and periods of extreme depression. Also called manic-depression.

black-box experiment   An attempt to analyze a structure or organism without being able to see inside it.

blood   The mixture of plasma, red and white cells, platelets, and other substances that flows through the body, carrying oxygen and nutrients to the cells and removing waste products.

blood-brain barrier   A physical and chemical barrier formed by the central nervous system that prevents chemicals in the bloodstream from entering the brain.

blood poisoning   A form of blood-borne disease usually caused by bacteria that live and grow in the blood vessels. Also called septicemia.

botanist   A scientist who specializes in the field of BOTANY.

botany   The study of plants, their usable products, and their environments.

broad-spectrum antibiotic   An antibiotic that can combat many types of bacteria.

bronchitis   An infection of the membrane that lines the lungs' bronchial tubes.

callus   A thick growth of plant or animal cells, usually over a wound or at a site that is subject to frequent pressure. Calluses also form when plant cells are grown in a laboratory.

calomel   A poisonous mix of mercury and chlorine, also called mercurous chloride, that once was used as a laxative and as a purgative. Calomel is now used as a fungicide and as a local antibiotic.

cancer   Abnormal, out-of-control cellular growths that often lead to the death of humans or animals.

capillaries   Slender blood vessels that join arteries to veins.

carbolic acid   A poisonous acid derived from coal tar that is used as an antiseptic and disinfectant.

carcinogen   A chemical or other substance that can trigger the development and growth of cancer.

cardiopulmonary resuscitation (CPR)   A lifesaving method for maintaining heartbeat and breathing.

cell   The basic units of structure and function in living things. Cells are the smallest units of life that can carry on the activities of life.

central nervous system   The brain and the spinal cord in vertebrate animals.

chemist   A scientist who studies chemicals and their interactions. Also, another term for pharmacist, used in the United Kingdom and former member nations of the British Empire.

chemotherapy   A method of treating diseases by using chemicals that have specific and direct effects on those diseases.

chicken pox   A contagious skin disease caused by the *varicella* virus.

chloroform   An early form of anesthetic.

cholera   A disease of the gastrointestinal tract that causes cramping, vomiting, diarrhea, and extreme weakness.

clinical depression   Any form of depression caused by a lack of neurotransmitters or a similar chemical imbalance in the brain.

clotting   The blood's process of forming plugs or scabs on the surface of wounds or within the body. Blood clots that form within blood vessels can lead to strokes, heart attacks, or other medical problems.

cocaine   A narcotic chemical that can be used as a painkiller and as a stimulant. Derived from the coca plant, cocaine is extremely addictive and is illegal except for some tightly regulated medical uses.

cocktail   In medicine, a mixture of drugs that is designed to overwhelm a particular disease.

codeine   A derivative of opium used to suppress coughs, relieve pain, and induce sleep. Like opium, codeine can be addictive.

compassionate investigational new drug   In the United States, an unapproved experimental drug that the FDA allows physicians to prescribe for certain extreme diseases when no other drugs are available.

conjugation   In biology, a form of reproduction in which two single-celled organisms join, share genetic information, and then separate.

conjunctivitis   An infection of the mucous membrane that covers the surface of the eye and the interior of the eyelid; also known as pinkeye.

constipation   An inability to empty the bowels, especially when there is not enough natural lubrication in the bowels to move material along.

consumption   *See* TUBERCULOSIS.

control group   Organisms (such as cells, plants, animals, or people) that researchers do not expose to chemicals or other factors that they are studying.

coronary artery   One of the blood vessels that supply blood to the tissues of the heart.

coronary atherosclerosis   A form of arteriosclerosis that affects the coronary arteries.

CPR   *See* CARDIOPULMONARY RESUSCITATION.

cytosine   One of the three chemical bases present in DNA and RNA.

daughter cell   One of the cells formed by cellular reproduction.

decay   To deteriorate or break down. Also, in physics, the disintegration of some elements through the loss of protons and neutrons, causing the element to change into another one.

deoxyribonucleic acid (DNA)   One form of genetic material that determines an organism's shape, function, and other characteristics. DNA molecules consist of long sequences of smaller units called nucleotides.

depression   A mental disorder marked by long periods of sadness and other negative feelings that is more serious than normal "down" moods.

dexfenfluramine   One of the two chemicals that made up the *fen* portion of the weight-loss drug FEN-PHEN.

diabetes   One of two diseases that are marked by the symptom of excessive urination. The most frequent kind of diabetes is diabetes mellitus, an inability to metabolize sugar properly. The other kind, diabetes insipidus, is the excessive elimination of water from the body by the kidneys.

diabetes mellitus   An inability of the body to metabolize sugar either because the body lacks insulin or because it does not properly react to insulin.

diarrhea   Usually, a symptom of an intestinal disease that includes frequent defecation and loose, watery stools.

DNA   *See* DEOXYRIBONUCLEIC ACID.

doctor   A person who has earned a doctoral degree, which indicates he or she has mastered the highest level of study in a particular field. By common usage, the title *Doctor* most often refers to someone who has earned a doctorate in medicine, dentistry, or another medical profession.

double-blind test   A test of a pharmaceutical drug in which neither the patient who takes the drug nor the physician who hands it out know what the drug is. Double-blind tests usually match the drug being studied with a harmless placebo.

dropsy   An abnormal collection of fluid in some tissues or cavities of the body. Also known as edema.

drug resistance   The invulnerability of some microbes to a drug that previously was able to kill or control them.

duct   In the body, a tube that carries some hormones or other chemicals from the glands that secrete them to the organs that use them.

dysentery   An intestinal disease that causes intense diarrhea with blood and mucus.

Echinacea purpurea   The scientific name of the purple coneflower. Many people take extracts of echinacea as a natural means of boosting the immune system to prevent or treat colds or other infections.

echocardiogram   An analysis of heart function by bouncing ultrasonic waves off the heart.

elixir   In pharmacology, a sweetened liquid containing alcohol mixed with a medicinal substance.

embryo   An infant in the earliest stages of development.

emetic   A substance that causes vomiting.

enamel   The hard material that covers the surface of the teeth.

endocrine system   The system of glands that secrete their hormones and other chemicals directly into the blood or lymph, rather than through a duct.

endorphin   One of the substances produced in the brain to suppress pain and control some physiological operations.

ephedra   One of several plants that produce ephedrine. The Chinese plant ma huang is a variety of ephedra.

ephedrine   An antiallergy drug, asthma, and hay fever drug derived from some varieties of the ephedra plant.

epidemic   The rapid spread of a disease through a community, a nation, or the world.

epidemiology   The study of epidemics, how they develop, and how to control them.

erythema nodosum laprosum (ENL)   A symptom of leprosy that causes painful sores and boils on the surface of the body.

erythrocyte   *See* RED BLOOD CELL.

Escherichia coli   A common intestinal bacteria that has been genetically engineered to produce insulin.

ether   A colorless, sweet-smelling liquid that evaporates quickly and is used as an anesthetic.

ethical medicine   A scientifically derived medicinal drug produced by professional pharmacists or pharmaceutical companies. This term was used to separate pharmaceuticals from patent medicines.

FDA   *See* FOOD AND DRUG ADMINISTRATION.

fenfluramine   One of the two chemicals that made up the *fen* portion of the weight-loss drug FEN-PHEN.

fen-phen   A popular weight-loss drug that was banned in many nations after it was found to cause heart damage.

fetus   An animal embryo in the later stages of its development.

fever   A condition in which the body's temperature is higher than normal. In humans, who have a normal temperature of roughly 98.6 degrees Fahrenheit (37 degrees centigrade), fevers of above

102 degrees Fahrenheit (38.9 degrees centigrade) are considered serious enough to be life threatening.

first aid   Emergency or immediate treatment for injury or illness.

flagellum   A whiplike appendage that a bacterium or other organism uses to move around.

flesh-eating disease   *See* NECROTIZING FASCIITIS.

flu shot   *See* INFLUENZA VACCINE.

Food and Drug Administration   An agency of the U.S. Department of Health and Human Services that oversees the development and production of drugs, biological products, and therapeutic devices. The FDA also is responsible for monitoring the purity of food produced or sold within the United States, the safety of cosmetics, and the proper packaging and labeling of all these products.

formulation   The chemical makeup of a medical drug.

Frankenfood   A nickname given to genetically modified foods by people who oppose them.

fungus   Any member of the biological kingdom called *fungi*, which are plantlike organisms that do not have leaves, flowers, or chlorophyll, and do not have the type of vascular system that plants use to absorb nutrients.

gastrointestinal tract   The portion of the alimentary canal that includes the stomach and the intestines.

gelatin   Any colorless, tasteless protein jelly.

gene   A sequence of nucleotide bases on a DNA molecule that determines the characteristics of living things.

generic drug   A nontrademarked form of a trademarked, brand-name drug. Under U.S. drug laws, generic drugs can contain as little as 80 percent of the active ingredients found in that medicine's brand-name form, provided the drug has the same effect as the original.

genetically modified   Any living organism, from cells to animals, whose genetic code has been artificially changed to introduce or eliminate one or more traits.

genome   The complete genetic sequence of a living creature.

germ   A microscopic organism, particularly one that causes a disease. *See also* MICROBE.

gestation   The time it takes an infant to develop from a fertilized egg to a living individual.

goiter   A swelling of the thyroid gland.

gonorrhea   An inflammation of the mucous membranes of the genitals and urinary tract caused by the sexually transmitted *Gonococcus* bacterium.

guanine One of the three chemical bases present in DNA and RNA.

guild An association of people who practice a similar trade.

half-life The time it takes half a sample of radioactive material to decay.

Hansen's disease *See* LEPROSY.

hardening of the arteries *See* ARTERIOSCLEROSIS.

heart murmur The noise caused by blood flowing backwards through a damaged heart valve.

helix A spiral shape, similar to the rails of a spiral staircase.

herbalist Someone who studies and practices the techniques of herbal medicine.

herbal medicine The practice of using plants and other natural materials to cure disease and heal other maladies.

herbal remedy An herb, a flower, or another plant that supposedly is able to treat a particular medical condition.

heroic medicine A form of Western medicine based on the idea that diseases needed to be treated with purgatives, emetics, and other extreme forms of medicine.

hiera picra A combination of herbs that served as both a purgative and a decongestant.

histamine A chemical the body releases in response to an allergen that lowers blood pressure and has other effects on the body.

HIV *See* HUMAN IMMUNODEFICIENCY VIRUS.

hormones Proteins produced by special glands within the body that regulate metabolic reactions in other cells.

hot flash A sudden feeling of heat sweeping over the body that women sometimes feel during menopause.

human immunodeficiency virus (HIV) A virus that attacks cells of the immune system and can lead to the development of AIDS.

humor One of the fluids that physicians and philosophers once thought controlled health and emotional disposition.

hybrid A genetic mixture of two different species.

hypodermic A needle designed to inject medicine under the skin. Also, a type of medicine designed to be placed under the skin.

immune system The assemblage of organs, tissues, and cells that detects and fights off diseases.

immunologist A scientist who studies the function of the immune system and how people become immune to diseases.

IND *See* INVESTIGATIONAL NEW DRUG.

indigestion An inability to digest or difficulty in digesting food that sometimes causes the body to produce excess stomach acid.

inert   In medicine and chemistry, something that has few, if any, chemical properties.

inert ingredients   The materials that contain a drug's active ingredients in a pill, a liquid, or an inhalant.

infantile paralysis   *See* POLIOMYELITIS.

influenza   An infectious viral disease caused by any of a number of strains of the influenza virus. Also called the flu.

influenza vaccine   A drug made from killed versions of the influenza virus that helps people ward off the flu.

inoculation   The injection of a substance into the body to create immunity. *See also* VACCINATION.

insane asylum   A hospital or other facility that was designed to treat or simply contain people with extreme mental illnesses.

insulin   A hormone that regulates the body's ability to absorb and process sugar.

Internet   A globe-spanning network of interconnected computer systems. Though it is the most well-known network, the Internet is actually just one of several networks that exist to help people exchange news and ideas with one another.

Investigational New Drug (IND)   A category of experimental drugs that is being put through a series of clinical trials in preparation for approval by the U.S. Food and Drug Administration.

in vitro   From a Latin phrase meaning "in glass," this term means something that is placed or grows in an artificial environment, such as a flask or a test tube.

in vivo   From a Latin phrase meaning "in life," this term means something that grows in a live organism.

jaundice   A yellowish discoloration of the skin and eyes that can be caused by liver disease, the breakdown of red blood cells, or a few other medical conditions.

laudanum   A mixture of water, alcohol, and opium that once was used as a painkiller.

laughing gas   *See* NITROUS OXIDE.

laxative   A medicine that helps the body evacuate the bowels.

leprosy   A wasting disease of the skin and nerves that can lead to muscle weakness and other problems. Also called Hansen's disease.

leukocyte   One of five types of blood cells that attack and destroy disease organisms. Also called white blood cells.

lymph   Excess body fluid that leaks out of the blood and body tissues and needs to be returned to the blood.

lymphatic system   The circulatory system that collects lymph and returns it to the blood.

magic bullet A drug that targets a particular disease with almost total success.

ma huang *See* EPHEDRA.

malaria A potentially fatal parasitic disease that causes alternating chills and fever, as well as anemia.

mania A type of mental illness that causes extreme levels of overactivity, euphoria, or irritability.

manic-depression *See* BIPOLAR DISORDER.

materia medica Literally, "the material of medicine." The drugs and other substances used in the practice of medicine, as well as the study of these materials.

MDR *See* MULTIPLE-DRUG-RESISTANT.

medicine The practice of treating disease, injuries, and other health problems. Also, a chemical used to treat diseases, pain, or other maladies.

medicine, heroic *See* HEROIC MEDICINE.

medicine man *See* SHAMAN.

medicine show A traveling group of performers whose acts are designed to sell a NOSTRUM or other patent medicine.

megadose An extremely large dose of medicine, vitamins, or other chemicals to treat or prevent illness.

mental illness An inability of the brain to properly regulate a person's moods, emotions, or perceptions of the world.

mercurous chloride *See* CALOMEL.

microbe A microscopic organism, particularly one that causes disease.

Middle Ages The historical period from the fall of the Western Roman Empire in roughly A.D. 500 to the spread of the Renaissance by A.D. 1450.

milk of magnesia A mix of water and the chemical magnesium hydroxide, used as a laxative.

mineral oil A laxative distilled from petroleum oil.

MAOI *See* MONOAMINE OXIDASE INHIBITOR.

mold A type of fungus that grows on food, in soil, and on other surfaces.

molecule A chemical unit made up of two or more atoms held together by sharing electrons.

monoamine oxidase inhibitor (MAOI) A type of antidepressant that prevents the body from forming a protein that breaks down neurotransmitters.

morphine An addictive painkiller derived from opium.

multiple-drug-resistant (MDR) A microbe that has evolved the ability to withstand a large number of antibiotics or other drugs to which it once was vulnerable.

mutation   A change in the genetic structure of an organism.

Mycobacterium tuberculosis   The bacterium that causes tuberculosis.

narcotic   A chemical such as morphine that numbs the central nervous system. Most narcotics have an analgesic, or painkilling, effect. Using narcotic analgesics carries the risk of addiction.

narcotic analgesic   *See* NARCOTIC.

necrotizing fasciitis   A skin disease caused by a strain of the *Streptococcus* bacterium. It is nicknamed the "flesh-eating disease" because the bacteria attacks and kills healthy skin cells as well as the cells of patients with compromised immune systems.

nervous system   The communication network that allows an animal's organs and other systems to regulate how they work and, in higher animals, connects these systems to the brain.

neuron   An individual nerve cell.

neurotransmitter   A chemical that neurons use to transmit signals to each other.

nitrous oxide   A gas used as an anesthetic. Also called laughing gas because of the feeling of giddiness it creates.

nonnarcotic analgesic   A painkiller such as aspirin or ibuprofen that prevents the body from forming prostaglandins. Using nonnarcotic analgesics does not pose any risk of addiction.

nonsteroidal anti-inflammatory drugs   Medicines such as aspirin and ibuprofen that reduce or eliminate swelling in injured tissues without using steroids.

nostrum   A medicine recommended by its maker or manufacturer without any scientific proof of its value or effectiveness.

nucleus   In biology, the structure in a cell that contains the cell's DNA.

nurse practitioner   A nurse who has had specialized training in one or more areas of medicine.

obese   More than 30 pounds overweight.

off-label use   The ability of physicians to prescribe any federally approved medicine to treat any medical condition that they judge the drug might help heal.

ointment   A medical cream usually made from oil or fat.

opium   A narcotic drug made from the sap of poppies.

opportunistic infection   A disease that establishes itself in someone whose immune system already is weakened by another infection.

organic farming   A farming method that does not include chemical fertilizers or insecticides.

orphan drug   A drug that treats a disease so rare that only a small number of people suffer from it.

osteoporosis A thinning or weakening of the bones that accompanies old age and some diseases.

OTC *See* OVER-THE-COUNTER MEDICINE.

over-the-counter medicine A pharmaceutical drug that can be sold without a prescription.

oxidation A form of chemical decay caused when a substance combines with oxygen.

paclitaxel A cancer-fighting drug that can be obtained from a few varieties of the yew tree.

parasite A plant or an animal that lives within and feeds on another living creature.

particle accelerator A device that hurls fast-moving streams of sub-atomic particles into each other or into atomic targets in order to study their structure. Also called atom smashers.

patent A government grant that gives people or companies the exclusive right to make and sell their inventions for a limited period.

patent medicine A generally useless, and often addicting, chemical compound that is sold as medicine with no proof that it actually works.

pathology The study of diseases, their causes, and their effects on the body.

PCP *See* PHENCYCLIDINE.

penicillin The first of the mold-derived antibiotics.

Penicillium notatum The mold that originally yielded the antibiotic penicillin.

peripheral nervous system The portion of the nervous system that runs from the central nervous system to the extremities.

petri dish A small, flat, circular dish, often with a cover, that is used to grow bacteria and other microbes.

pharmaceutical A medicinal drug, or something that involves the preparation or use of medicinal drugs.

pharmacist A professional chemist who is licensed to sell drugs and prepare prescriptions. Pharmacists may also specially mix, or compound, drugs in their own laboratories.

pharmacologist A scientist who searches for new drugs, studies their safety and efficacy, and determines the best way to manufacture them.

pharmacology The scientific study of how drugs affect living things.

pharmacopoeia An official list of standard drugs, their preparation, and their usage.

pharmacy The profession of preparing, distributing, and selling drugs. Also, a store that prepares and/or sells drugs.

phencyclidine (PCP) A powerful depressant that legally is used only as an elephant and monkey tranquilizer. Also called angel dust because of its hallucinogenic effect in humans.

phentermine The chemical that made up the *phen* portion of the weight-loss drug FEN-PHEN.

phlegm Mucus produced by the nose, throat, and lungs as a reaction to colds or other illnesses.

physician A licensed doctor of medicine.

"the Pill" A birth-control drug that uses female hormones to alter a woman's reproductive cycle.

pituitary gland An endocrine gland that helps control growth, regulates the metabolism, and performs other functions.

placebo effect A tendency of people to recover from an illness or to stop feeling pain simply by taking a pill, whether or not it contains any medicine.

placebo test A method of testing the effectiveness of a proposed medicine by giving the drug to one group of volunteers and giving a placebo to another group.

plague One of a number of devastating diseases caused by the bacteria *Yersinia pestis*.

pneumonia Any disease that causes an inflammation of the lungs.

polio The common term for POLIOMYELITIS.

poliomyelitis A viral infection of the brain and spinal column that can lead to partial paralysis, total paralysis, or death.

poultice A soft, moist mass of substances (such as herbs or chemicals) applied to the body to treat infections or injuries.

pox A disease that covers the body with pus-filled sores.

preclinical testing Laboratory and animal tests that determine whether a chemical can treat a particular disease effectively and safely enough to test it on human volunteers.

prescription A written order from a physician or a dentist to dispense drugs to a patient.

prescription drug A drug that can be dispensed only with a physician's or a dentist's written order.

priests' bitters *See* HIERA PICRA.

prostaglandin A hormonelike substance that seems to help nerve cells carry messages about pain sensations, among other effects.

protease inhibitor A class of anti-AIDS drugs that block one of the stages of HIV reproduction.

protozoa Plural form of the word *protozoan*.

protozoan A one-celled organism that contains its genetic material within a separate nucleus.

pseudoephedrine   A cold and allergy medicine that is similar to ephedrine.

psychopharmacological   A chemical that has an effect on the chemistry of the brain.

psychopharmacology   A branch of pharmacology that deals with drugs that can affect brain chemistry.

psychosis   A severe form of mental illness that can include hallucinations and delusions.

purgative   Something that causes the bowels to empty.

purge   To rid the body of poisons or other unwanted substances by vomiting or bleeding.

purple coneflower   *See ECHINACEA PURPUREA.*

quack medicine   A useless or fraudulent drug or medical technique.

quinine   An anti-malaria drug derived from the cinchona plant.

rabies   A viral infection of the central nervous system that causes mental disturbances and muscular paralysis.

radioactive decay   The breakdown of some elements into other forms through the loss of subatomic particles.

receptor   A molecule or group of molecules on a cell that is designed to receive a particular protein or other chemical.

recombinant DNA   A method of inserting part of the DNA of one organism into the genetic code of another.

red blood cell   *See ERYTHROCYTE.*

Renaissance   A cultural and intellectual movement that started in Italy in the 14th century A.D. and spread to the rest of Europe by the late 15th century, ending the historic period called the Middle Ages.

Reye's syndrome   A rare form of potentially fatal childhood brain damage that can come from taking aspirin during a viral infection.

ribonucleic acid (RNA)   A chemical within living cells that plays a central role in the formation of proteins.

risk group   The portion of a population that is most likely to develop a disease.

RNA   *See RIBONUCLEIC ACID.*

Rocky Mountain spotted fever   An often fatal disease that causes fevers, chills, and rashes. It is caused by a type of bacteria called *Rickettsias* that are spread by the bite of the Rocky Mountain wood tick and the American dog tick.

sacred bitters   *See HIERA PICRA.*

SAD   *See SEASONAL AFFECTIVE DISORDER.*

Saint-John's-wort   An herb that is thought to contain a natural antidepressant.

salicylic acid   A chemical in the bark of the willow plant that acts as a headache and fever cure.

Salvarsan   An arsenic-based drug that served as a MAGIC BULLET against the sexually transmitted disease syphilis.

scarlet fever   A disease caused by a type of *Streptococcus* bacteria that causes bright-red rashes and mainly strikes children.

schizophrenia   A severe mental disease that prevents its victims from thinking and reacting realistically.

scientific method   The process of explaining natural phenomena through observation, hypothesis, and experimentation. The scientific method also involves verification of one's work by other scientists.

seasonal affective disorder (SAD)   A form of depression many people develop during the winter or at other times of reduced daylight.

selective serotonin reuptake inhibitor (SSRI)   A type of antidepressant that prevents nerve cells in the brain from reabsorbing a neurotransmitter called serotonin.

semisynthetic   A drug or other substance that comes from the chemical processing of natural materials.

septicemia   *See* BLOOD POISONING.

sequence   The pattern of amino acids in DNA or RNA.

sequencing   Determining the sequence of bases and the genes they encode in a molecule of DNA or RNA.

shaman   A tribal healer who combines mystical and physical practices, including herbal medical techniques, to treat illness.

shock treatment   A method of treating mental illness by the controlled electrocution of the brain.

sickle-cell anemia   An inherited condition in which red blood cells form in crescent shapes, rather than in their normal disks.

side effect   A reaction to a drug that does not have any effect on the disease or condition being treated.

signed plants   Plants that supposedly contained the power to heal the body parts they resembled.

simples   Herbs or other plants that were used as medicines.

spirochetes   A group of spiral-shaped bacteria, one of which causes syphilis.

sponsor   An individual, a company, or an agency that submits a request to test a drug on human volunteers.

SSRI   *See* SELECTIVE SEROTONIN REUPTAKE INHIBITOR.

Staphylococcus   A type of bacteria responsible for many diseases and skin conditions.

stem cell   A primitive cell that can develop into a number of specialized cells.

strain In biology, a particular type of organism within a species or a subspecies.

Streptococcus A type of bacteria responsible for many infections, such as sinus infections, tooth decay, ear infections, and blood poisoning.

sulfa drugs A group of drugs that include the chemical sulfur dioxide in their chemical makeup and halt the growth of some types of bacteria.

sulfanilamide The first of the sulfa drugs to receive widespread use against infections.

synapse In biology, the gap between two or more nerve cells.

synthesize To make a substance or an element in a laboratory.

TB *See* TUBERCULOSIS.

terra sigillata A type of soft, clay-rich soil that supposedly could neutralize poisons and calm disorders of the stomach and intestines. Also known as "sealed earth" because packages of it were stamped with the symbol of the islands from which they came.

theriac An all-purpose, supposedly medicinal syrup that was commonly used until the 19th century.

thymine A chemical base present in DNA but not RNA.

toxin A poison secreted by a living organism.

transgene A segment of an organism's genetic code that has been transferred to another organism.

transgenic Containing genes that have been transplanted from another organism.

transgenic animal An organism that has been genetically modified with genes from another organism.

treatment IND *See* COMPASSIONATE INVESTIGATIONAL NEW DRUG.

tricyclic antidepressant A type of antidepressant that prevents nerve cells in the brain from reabsorbing a number of neurotransmitters.

trypanosome A parasitic, single-celled organism that causes sleeping sickness and other diseases.

tuberculosis An infectious, bacteria-caused lung disease that has become resistant to many antibiotics. Formerly known as consumption.

typhoid fever An extremely infectious bacterial disease that causes fever, weakness, and death.

undifferentiated cell *See* STEM CELL.

United States Federal Trade Commission (FTC) The federal government agency that regulates advertising and other trade matters.

United States Pharmacopoeia (U.S.P.) The book that establishes standards for drugs and drug products in the United States.

uracil   A chemical BASE present in RNA but not DNA.

U.S.P.   *See* UNITED STATES PHARMACOPOEIA.

vaccination   The process of making people immune to diseases through inoculation.

vaccine   A dead or weakened disease organism that triggers a body's immune system to make antibodies against that disease.

vein   A blood vessel that carries blood back to the heart.

vestibular apparatus   A section of the inner ear that helps people keep their balance and determine their direction of motion.

virus   An extremely small, extremely simple infectious agent that can grow and duplicate itself only in a living cell. Typically, a virus is little more than a core of DNA or RNA surrounded by a shell of protein that can chemically open the wall of the virus's normal host cell.

vitamin   A nutrient that the body needs in small amounts in order to function properly.

white blood cell   *See* LEUKOCYTE.

wise woman   In the Middle Ages and the Renaissance, a woman who knew the healing powers of plants and how to use them.

World Wide Web   A subset of the Internet that presents information in an easy-to-read form, often using colors and graphics. Web pages can be connected via *hyperlinks.*

worms   In medicine, long, multicellular parasites that infest the gastrointestinal tract.

yang   In Chinese philosophy, the energy force that represents light, heat, and activity. See also YIN.

yellow fever   A viral disease that causes high fevers, jaundice, and bleeding.

yin   In Chinese philosophy, the energy force that represents darkness, cold, and passivity. See also YANG.

zygote   A fertilized egg.

FURTHER READING

Bernstein, Leslie. "Dementia without a Cause." *Discover* 21, no. 2 (February 2000): 104.

Burger, Alfred. *Drugs and People: Medications, Their History and Origins, and the Way They Act.* Charlottesville: University Press of Virginia, 1986.

Christensen, Damaris. "Medical Mimicry." *Science News* 159, no. 5 (February 3, 2001): 74–78.

Clifford, Lee. "Tyrannosaurus Rx." *Fortune* 142, no. 10 (October 30, 2000): 140–150.

Cohen, Jon. "Consulting Biotech's Oracle." *Technology Review* 104, no. 8 (October 2001): 70–76.

Cowen, David L., and William H. Helfand. *Pharmacy: An Illustrated History.* New York: Abrams, 1990.

"The Debate over Stem Cells Gets Hot." *Discover* 23, no. 1 (January 2001): 56.

Duncan, David Ewing. "The Protein Hunters." *Wired* 9, no. 4 (April 2001): 164–171.

Fackelmann, Kathleen. "Medicine for Menopause." *Science News* 153, no. 25 (June 20, 1998): 392–393.

Fenster, J. M. "How Nobody Invented Anesthesia." *Invention & Technology* 12, no. 1 (Summer 1996): 24–35.

———. "The Conquest of Diabetes." *Invention & Technology* 14, no. 3 (winter 1999): 48–55.

Fox, Cynthia. "Why Stem Cells Will Transform Medicine." *Fortune* 143, no. 12 (June 11, 2001): 158–166.

Frist, Bill. *When Every Moment Counts: What You Need to Know about Bioterrorism from the Senate's Only Doctor.* Lanham, Md.: Rowman & Littlefield Publishers, 2002.

Gibbs, W. Wayt. "All in the Mind." *Scientific American* 285, no. 4 (October 2001): 16.

Glausiusz, Josie. "The Ice Man Healeth" *Discover* 21, no. 2 (February 2000): 16.

Hopkin, Karen. "The Post-Genome Project." *Scientific American* 265, no. 2 (August 2001): 16.

Jegalian, Karin. "The Gene Factory." *Technology Review* 102, no. 2 (March/April 1999): 64–68.

Jonietz, Erika. "Healthy Snacks." *Technology Review* 104, no. 4 (May 2001): 43.

Kessler, David A. and Karyn L. Feiden. "Faster Evaluation of Vital Drugs." *Scientific American* 272, no. 3 (March 1995): 48–54.

Lemley, Brad. "Alternative Medicine Man." *Discover* 20, no. 8 (August 1999): 56–63.

Masson, Terrence. *CG 101: A Computer Graphics Industry Reference.* Indianapolis, Ind.: New Riders Publishing, 1999.

"Medicine's Manhattan Project." *Technology Review* 102, no. 4 (July/August 1999): 96.

McClintock, Jack. "Blood Suckers." *Discover* 22, no. 12 (December 2001): 56–61.

Mestel, Rosie. "Drugs from the Sea." *Discover* 20, no. 3 (March 1999): 70–74.

Mlot, Christine. "Historical Cache of Medicinal Plants." *Science News* 151, no. 14 (April 5, 1997): 207.

Morton, Oliver. "Gene Machine." *Wired* 4, no. 7 (July 2001): 148–159.

Musto, David F. "Opium, Cocaine and Marijuana in American History." *Scientific American* 265, no. 1 (July 1991): 40–47.

Nalick, Jon. "Natural Wonders." *USC Health* 9, no. 2 (winter 2002): 14–15. Available online. URL: http://www.usc.edu/hsc/info/pr/hmm/hmm.html.

Nicholson, Rob. "AZ-Tech Medicine." *Natural History* 108, no. 10 (December 1999–January 2000): 54–59.

Oldstone, Michael B. A. *Viruses, Plagues, and History.* New York: Oxford University Press, 1998.

Parascandola, John. *The Development of American Pharmacology: John J. Abel and the Shaping of a Discipline.* Baltimore, Md.: Johns Hopkins University Press, 1992.

Perkins, Beth, and Misha Gravenor. "Adult Stem Cells." *Technology Review* 104, no. 9 (November 2001): 42–49.

Peterson, Ivars. "Computation Takes a Quantum Leap." *Science News* 158, no. 9 (August 26, 1997): 132.

Potera, Carol. "Making Needles Needless." *Technology Review* 101, no. 5 (September/October 1998): 66–70.

Preston, Richard. *The Hot Zone: A Terrifying True Story.* New York: Random House, 1994.

Radestsky, Peter. "The Last Days of the Wonder Drugs." *Discover* 19, no. 11 (November 1998): 74–85.

———. "The Good Virus." *Discover* 17, no. 11 (November 1996): 50–58.

Regaldo, Antonio. "Cures on Hold." *Technology Review* 103, no. 4 (August 2000): 30.

———. "The Great Gene Grab." *Technology Review* 103, no. 5 (September/October 2000): 48–55.

———. "Mining the Genome." *Technology Review* 102, no. 5 (September/October 1999): 56–63.

Selim, Jocelyn. "Digging for Cures." *Discover* 21, no. 12 (December 2000): 28.

Seppa, Nathan. "Bacteria Provide a Frontline Defense." *Science News* 158, no. 16 (October 14, 2000): 244.

Shapiro, Robert. *The Human Blueprint: The Race to Unlock the Secrets of Our Genetic Script.* New York: St. Martin's Press, 1991.

Smaglik, Paul. "Proliferation of Pills." *Science News* 151, no. 20 (May 17, 1997): 310–311.

Stephens, Trent, and Rock Brynner. *Dark Remedy: The Impact of Thalidomide and Its Revival as a Vital Medicine.* Cambridge, Mass.: Perseus Publishing, 2001.

Stikeman, Alexandra. "Calling All PCs." *Technology Review* 104, no. 4 (May 2001): 33.

———. "The Programmable Pill." *Technology Review* 104, no. 4 (May 2001): 78–83.

Stipp, David. "A Pill to Help You Remember." *Fortune* 144, no. 9 (November 12, 2001): 162–172.

"St. John's Wort Ineffective for Depression, Study Finds." *ScienceDaily Magazine*, Wednesday, April 10, 2002. Available on-line. URL: http://www.sciencedaily.com/releases/2002/04/020410075818.htm.

Swerdlow, Joel L. "Nature's Rx." *National Geographic* 197, no. 4 (April 2000): 98–117.

Taubes, Gary. "Antibody Revival." *Technology Review* 105, no. 6 (July/August 2002): 56–65.

———. "The Cold Warriors." *Discover* 20, no. 2 (February 1999): 40–50.

———. "Speeding Drug Discovery." *Technology Review* 104, no. 8 (October 2001): 62–69.

Thieme, Trevor. "A Pill with Your Name on It." *Discover* 22, no. 12 (December 2001): 28–29.

Trachtman, Paul. "Open Wide and Say 'Alternative Medicine.'" *Smithsonian* 25, no. 6 (September 1994): 110–123.

Travis, John. "Biological Warfare." *Science News* 149, no. 22 (June 1, 1996): 350–351.

———. "Human Embryonic Stem Cells Found?" *Science News* 152, no. 3 (July 19, 1997): 36.

———. "Viruses That Slay Bacteria Draw New Interest." *Science News* 157, no. 23 (June 3, 2000): 358.

Werth, Barry. *The Billion Dollar Molecule: One Company's Quest for the Perfect Drug.* New York: Simon & Schuster, 1994.

Whitlock, Chuck. *MediScams: How to Spot and Avoid Health Care Scams, Medical Frauds, and Quackery from the Local Physician to the Major Health Care Providers and Drug Manufacturers.* Los Angeles, Calif.: Renaissance Books, 2001.

Wright, Karen. "Thalidomide Is Back." *Discover* 21, no. 4 (April 2000): 31–33.

Zacks, Rebecca. "Custom-Made Medications." *Technology Review* 104, no. 10 (December 2001): 82–85.

———. "Under Biology's Hood." *Technology Review* 104, no. 7 (September 2001): 53–57.

"Who Killed the Iceman?" *National Geographic* 201, no. 2 (February 2002): 98–117.

WORLD WIDE WEB SITES

The following list is a sample of sites on the World Wide Web that provide information on modern medicines. The list includes government health information sources, a few of the world's top pharmaceutical companies, and some related independent organizations. The addresses for these sites were current as of May 2003; owing to the nature of the Internet and the rapid changes that can take place there, however, they may have changed after this book was published. If so, and if the site has not gone out of business, the new addresses might be found by searching the Web for the site's name. Otherwise, running a search for terms used in this book—such as *pharmaceuticals, pharmacology, medicine,* or *drug research*—should yield enough information to satisfy anyone's curiosity.

Government Health Information Sites

1. U.S. Food and Drug Administration: http://www.fda.gov
2. U.S. Department of Health and Human Services: http://www.hhs.gov
3. Healthfinder, a site maintained by the Department of Health and Human Services that provides links to health information: http://www.healthfinder.gov
4. www.health.gov, another Health and Human Services site with links to government health information and programs: http://www.health.gov
5. National Institutes of Health: http://www.nih.gov and http://www.health.nih.gov

6. National Center for Complementary and Alternative Medicine, a part of the National Institutes of Health: http://nccam.nih.gov
7. Centers for Disease Control and Prevention: http:/www.cdc.gov
8. Health Canada Online, a Web site operated by Health Canada, the federal department that serves as Canada's central health agency: http://www.hc-sc.gc.ca
9. The National Health Service of the United Kingdom: http://www.nhs.uk
10. The World Health Organization: http://www.who.int/en

Independent Organizations

1. U.S. Pharmacopeia, the organization that maintains the standards for pharmaceutical drugs in the United States: http://www.usp.org
2. American Chemical Society, a professional association for scientists who work in all fields of chemistry and associated sciences: http://www.acs.org
3. American Medical Association, the nation's best-known professional group for medical practitioners: http://www.ama-assn.org
4. American Association of Pharmaceutical Scientists, an organization that promotes knowledge of and research into medicinal drugs: http://www.aaps.org

Pharmaceutical History

1. The Pharmaceutical Century, a comprehensive history of pharmaceuticals in the 20th century prepared by the American Chemical Society: http://pubs.acs.org/journals/pharmcent/index.html
2. American Institute of the History of Pharmacy, a nonprofit group located at the University of Wisconsin: http://www.pharmacy.wisc.edu/aihp
3. The History of Medicine Division of the National Institutes for Health's National Library of Medicine: http://www.nlm.nih.gov/hmd/hmd.html

Selected Pharmaceutical Companies

1. Bayer Corporation, the company that first marketed aspirin as a prescription drug and later as an over-the-counter medication: http://www.bayer.com
2. Bristol-Myers Squibb Company, the company that manufactures paclitaxel under the Taxol brand name: http://www.bms.com

3. Eli Lilly and Company, the drug manufacturer that pioneered the production of insulin in the United States and is one of the leading pharmaceutical houses: http://www.lilly.com
4. Genentech, Inc., one of the leading companies that specializes in genetically engineered pharmaceuticals: http://www.gene.com
5. Johnson & Johnson, a pharmaceutical and medical equipment company that is involved in nearly every aspect of health care: http://www.jnj.com
6. Merck & Company, Inc., one of the world's premier drug research and manufacturing corporations: http://www.merck.com
7. Pharmacia, formerly the Upjohn Company: http://www.pnu.com

In addition, the Virtual Library's pharmacy Web site has a page of links to many other pharmaceutical companies at http://www.pharmacy.org/company.html.

Other Sites

1. PharmWeb, an Internet service that specializes in providing information on pharmaceuticals and other health topics: http://www.pharmweb.net
2. Library of the National Medical Association, an online reference source for health care professionals and the public: http://www.medical-library.org
3. Quackwatch, a Web site maintained by a nationally recognized physician who seeks to expose faulty or fraudulent medical practices: http://www.quackwatch.org

INDEX

Italic page numbers indicate illustrations.